Improving
Your Memory

Improving Your Memory

How to Remember What You're Starting to Forget

THIRD EDITION

Janet Fogler and
Lynn Stern

The Johns Hopkins University Press
Baltimore and London

The Johns Hopkins University Press
2715 North Charles Street
Baltimore, Maryland 21218-4363
www.press.jhu.edu

Library of Congress Cataloging-in-Publication Data

Fogler, Janet.
    Improving your memory : how to remember what you're starting to forget /
Janet Fogler and Lynn Stern — 3rd ed.
        p. cm.
ISBN 0-8018-8116-1 (pbk. : alk. paper)
1. Memory in old age. 2. Memory—Age factors. 3. Mnemonics. I. Stern, Lynn,
1949–   II. Title.
BF724.85.M45F64 2005
155.67'1314—dc22   2004025486

A catalog record for this book is available from the British Library.

Contents

IV Techniques for Improving Your Memory

Acknowledgments

We would like to express our appreciation and gratitude to all of our colleagues at the University of Michigan Health Systems, especially Ruth Campbell. Thanks also to Scott and Neal for their good humor and support.

I How Memory Works

1 You Can Improve Your Memory

EXAMPLES

Louise has a busy schedule as a clerk in a toy store and as an active grandmother. She's good at her job and never misses a grandchild's soccer game. Recently, she was shocked when she ran into an acquaintance at a soccer game and could not call her by name. A week later Louise walked out of the shopping mall and couldn't remember where she had parked her car. The following month, she realized she was losing track of the cast of characters in a novel she was reading. Then she completely forgot a lunch date with a good friend. Louise was extremely worried, especially when she thought of her uncle, who had been diagnosed with Alzheimer's disease.

Tom is retired from his job as an engineer and fills his schedule with volunteer work. Recently, he couldn't remember if he had changed the oil in his car the previous month or just thought about doing it. He missed the turn to the recreation center and didn't realize it until several streets later. He hid a house key in the garage and couldn't remember where. Tom checked with his doctor to see whether there was a medical reason for his forgetfulness.

You or your friends may have had experiences similar to Tom's and Louise's, and you, too, may have concerns about your memory. People of all ages complain about forgetting, but older people often worry about getting Alzheimer's disease when they cannot remember a cousin's name or where they put their keys. Memory does change as people grow older, but for almost everyone, memory can be improved with training and practice.

Here are some common complaints that we have heard from older people. (We need to confess that we have made these statements, too!)

- I went into a room and couldn't remember why.
- I couldn't remember what I wanted to ask the doctor.
- I forgot whether I'd taken my medication.
- I put my necklace away and can't remember where.
- I had to pay a late fee because I didn't pay the electric bill on time.
- I forgot to bring my camera on a trip.
- I went to the store for milk and got everything but.
- I forgot my sister's birthday.

If you have had any of these experiences, you can benefit from this book. We will teach you how to avoid common memory failures.

No one can remember everything. We all must make choices about what we want to remember and then put effort into areas that are most important to us. Over a lifetime you have acquired a pool of information from both educational and everyday experiences. These experiences have produced a wisdom that allows you to determine what new information is important for you to remember.

In this book we will help you make choices about where to put your memory effort, based on an understanding of how memory works and how it changes with age. We will also describe concrete strategies you can use to tackle the areas of memory that trouble you most.

To make this information more meaningful, we include many examples from daily life. Pen-and-paper exercises demonstrate memory concepts and techniques. Completing the assignments will help you improve your ability to remember the important things you may be starting to forget.

You will find this book most helpful if you read it carefully, do all the exercises, and use the suggestions in your daily life. We can't promise that you will never forget anything ever again, but we know that you can make positive changes in your memory and have fun doing it.

2   Understanding the Components of Memory

If you frequently say, "I just can't remember anymore!" or "My memory has gotten so bad!" you may have given in to the myth that aging and memory loss go hand in hand. Believing this myth keeps many people from even trying to remember. But we know that memory can be improved with training and practice.

To improve the memory process, it helps to understand how memory works. Although the brain is not understood nearly as well as the heart or the circulatory system, memory experts have devised a way to visualize how we remember. They often describe the memory process as having three components.

1. **Sensory memory,** the first component of the memory process, is the mind's brief recognition of what we see, hear, touch, smell, or taste. We are constantly surrounded by sights and sounds, and much of what we see and hear is discarded immediately. There is no need for us to record it. When we pay attention to a sensory impression, however, it enters the second component of memory, known as "working memory."

2. **Working memory** may be equated with conscious thought: the small amount of material that can be held in the mind at any given moment. Most experts believe that working memory can hold no more than six or seven items. This mate-

6

rial will be discarded in five to ten seconds unless it is either continually repeated or stored in long-term memory.

An example of information that is held in working memory and generally discarded without being stored is a seven-digit telephone number. When you look up a phone number, close the phone book, dial the number, and get a busy signal, you often realize that you've already forgotten the number you just dialed. This is a good demonstration of how briefly information is held in working memory. In another instance, you may hear a nutritionist say that there are eleven grams of fat in one tablespoon of butter. You are surprised at how high this number is. Later, however, you can't recall or even recognize the exact number. As you read this book, keep in mind this important fact—not all information that registers in working memory gets stored in long-term memory.

3. **Long-term memory,** the memory bank, is the largest component of the memory system. Its storage space is practically limitless. A common misconception is that long-term memory refers to events that occurred a long time ago. In fact, long-term memory holds information that was learned as recently as a few minutes ago and as long ago as many decades. This storage space holds items as varied as

- your name
- what happened an hour ago
- where you spent last Thanksgiving
- the information needed to drive a car
- an image of your first-grade teacher
- the multiplication tables

Thus, long-term memory refers to any information that is no longer in conscious thought but is stored for potential recollection.

A MODEL FOR HOW MEMORY WORKS
The flow of information through the three stages of memory

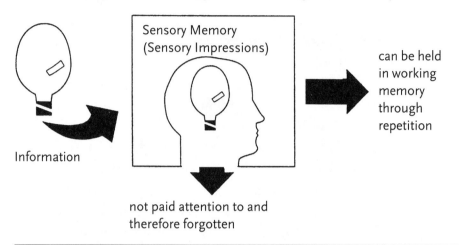

Sensory Memory
(Sensory Impressions)

can be held
in working
memory
through
repetition

Information

not paid attention to and
therefore forgotten

Here are two examples of how the memory process works in daily life.

EXAMPLES

You are doing your weekly shopping at the local grocery store. There are many items on the shelves that make sensory impressions on you. You see the colors of the packages, smell the bakery products, and hear the many sounds going on around you. These sensory impressions, however, may or may not register in conscious thought.

You pause in the produce department and consider what fruit is in season at this time of year. You glance at a papaya, a fruit you have never tried, and notice that it is very expensive. If you then move on, you will probably not recall the papaya in any detail. The impression of the papaya has entered working memory or conscious thought but has not necessarily been stored in long-term memory.

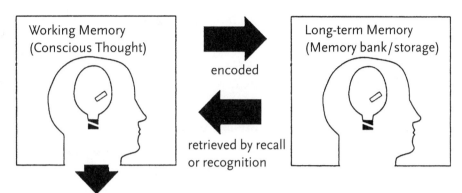

Working Memory
(Conscious Thought)

encoded

Long-term Memory
(Memory bank/storage)

retrieved by recall
or recognition

not transferred to long-term
memory and therefore forgotten

If you pay more attention to the papaya, however, by noting its shape, color, and texture, smelling its fragrance, feeling its ripeness, and even thinking about what it might taste like or how you could prepare it, the image and knowledge of that fruit will probably be transferred into long-term memory. This information will be available for retrieval in the future, for example, when you see a recipe that includes papaya as an ingredient.

You are addressing envelopes announcing the church bazaar. You have a list of names but no addresses. Your task is to look up the names in the phone book and transfer the addresses to the envelopes. As you handle the phone book, your senses take in the feel of the book, the faint smell of the ink, the pattern of the names on a given page, and the sound of pages turning, but these sensory impressions may or may not register in conscious thought.

You find Florence Tillman's name in the phone book and copy her address to an envelope: 4276 Woodlawn St., Chelsea,

Michigan. This information has entered working memory. You hold it in your mind for the few seconds needed to address the envelope. If you are not familiar with this street, you are unlikely to store this information in long-term memory. After a few moments, you probably won't even remember the name of the street.

If you note that Woodlawn Street is in your sister's neighborhood, however, and wonder whether your sister knows Ms. Tillman, you are more likely to transfer the information to long-term memory and think of Ms. Tillman as you drive down Woodlawn on the way to your sister's house.

Even though we have presented the components of memory as if new information always flows from sensory memory to working memory to long-term memory, it is possible for information that has not registered in conscious thought to be stored in long-term memory. In certain situations you may remember things without realizing that they have entered your awareness. For example, you may not be consciously aware of all of the people sitting in the doctor's waiting room with you, but when a man comes in and asks if you have seen a woman in a wheelchair, you recall that the nurse took a woman in a wheelchair into an exam room.

Now that you have learned about how memory works, you have a framework for recognizing why you may remember or forget certain things. Throughout the book, additional information, such as factors that affect memory and techniques to improve memory, will be related to this chapter that has described the components of the memory process.

3 How We Remember

Remembering depends on learning and storing information so that it can be retrieved at some future time. Thus, successful remembering requires

1. getting information solidly into long-term memory (this is called "encoding") and
2. bringing needed information from long-term memory into working memory (this is called "retrieval").

Let's discuss what is involved in these two aspects of the process of memory.

Encoding

The term "encoding" describes the process of getting information into long-term memory. Encoding consists of mental tasks, such as paying attention to something, associating it with something already known, analyzing the information for meaning, and elaborating on the details. Often these tasks are performed automatically, without any conscious effort on our part. These tasks give deeper meaning to the information and strengthen our chances of remembering it. Perhaps the easiest way to understand encoding is to look at how it works in the following examples.

EXAMPLES

Mrs. Yang is a confirmed people watcher. She loves to sit on a park bench and observe life around her. On any given day, she is aware of many people in the park walking their dogs. One day a puppy came up and licked her leg. She petted him, felt his soft fur, and enjoyed his exuberance. She asked the owner about the puppy's name and breed. She watched as the puppy explored the riverside area. Several days later, when she read a story about a puppy to her grandson, she recalled her day in the park and told him about the puppy. She was surprised that she remembered the puppy's name and breed so clearly. Although she had no recollection of the many other dogs she had seen that day, the information about the puppy had been well encoded because she had been interested, had paid attention, and had elaborated on the details of the interaction.

On another day in the park, Mrs. Yang sat next to a friendly woman about her age. After sharing a warm conversation, her new friend introduced herself as Mrs. Meadors. Mrs. Yang thought to herself, "I wish I could remember her name as well as I remember the name of the cute puppy I met." Instead of assuming that she couldn't do it, she decided to give it some thought and see if she could figure out a way to remember it. When she discovered that Mrs. Meadors grew up on a farm, she thought, "I can picture her in a meadow, which sounds like Meadors." In this example, Mrs. Yang intentionally encoded the information by paying attention to it, analyzing it, and associating it with something already known.

Two tasks of encoding—attention and association—deserve some additional emphasis.

Attention

Remember when your mother used to tell you to "pay attention." She was right! Paying attention, the first step in the process of encoding information into long-term memory, is one of the tasks of working memory. At any given moment, there are many pieces of information competing for the attention of your working memory. You may need to make a conscious effort to focus your attention on what you want to remember. Keep in mind that the amount of material you can hold in your working memory is quite limited. You need to zero in on what is important. The following examples may remind you of a time when your attention wasn't focused properly.

EXAMPLES

A friend tells you to meet her for lunch at 12:00, and you make a note of the date, time, and place in your appointment book. You mistakenly arrive at the restaurant at 12:30 because you didn't pay particular attention when the time was discussed, and you wrote it down incorrectly. Next time, resolve to focus your attention on the details of time and place, and be sure you write them down correctly.

You were given directions to a new dentist's office, followed them carefully, and had no trouble finding it the first time. At the next visit, you assume that you will remember where to go. As you approach the area, you realize that you don't know which high-rise building the office is in. What has happened is that you didn't pay enough attention to the location and the appearance of the building when you first saw it. In the future, note some landmarks and descriptive features that will differentiate one building from the next.

In both of these examples, you believed that you were paying enough attention to encode the information sufficiently, but clearly you weren't. Everyone has had this experience many times. We give superficial attention to a piece of information and then are frustrated when we can't remember it exactly. One of the simplest ways to improve your memory is to realize the importance of focusing your attention on what you really want to remember.

Since there are often many pieces of information competing for your attention, you may find that you have paid attention to the wrong thing and have missed what you really wanted to remember. For example, you're attending classes on memory improvement. All of a sudden you realize that you've been staring at a woman's unusual clothing instead of paying attention to the teacher. The next day you can still recall the purple sequined sweater with red sweat pants but have no recollection of the homework assignment. Focusing attention on what you really want to remember is a first step in improving memory. In the future, when you forget, ask yourself if the problem was inadequate attention.

Association

Another aspect of encoding that deserves some explanation is association. Whether we are aware of it or not, new information is encoded by connecting it with other well-known and relevant information already in long-term memory. This process is called "association." The easiest way to understand the concept of association is to look at how it happens effortlessly in daily life.

EXAMPLES

If you meet a new person, your memory of him may be encoded by making different associations. You may note what he looks like, where you met him, where he lives, what kind of work he does, and any friends you have in common. Thus, an association could be made with these different classifications: curly-haired people, the theater where you met, other people who live in his neighborhood, the medical profession, or the woman who introduced him to you. In the future, thinking of any of these categories could trigger a recollection of your new acquaintance. When you see another curly-haired person or a doctor or when you go to the theater, the experience may serve as a cue, and you may think of your new acquaintance.

Suppose your granddaughter has recently been chosen to be on the high-school field-hockey team. You don't know anything about how the game is played or the equipment that's used, but you do know a lot about football. When your granddaughter explains the game and equipment to you, you automatically associate the new information about field size, scoring, timekeeping, and protective equipment with what you already know about football. Without any such associations, information about field hockey would be difficult to encode. The next time you watch football on TV, you may think of your conversation with your granddaughter and remember that she has a field-hockey game coming up.

Much association of new information is done unconsciously, but you can make a conscious effort to associate something you want to remember with something you already know. The more effort you put into creating these associations and the greater the number of cross-references available, the more likely you are to recall at will. Here are two examples of people who have made a conscious effort to associate something they want to remember with something they know well.

EXAMPLES

Amir's granddaughter is fascinated by the children's TV show *Sesame Street.* He recently bought a book for her about many of the Sesame Street characters. When she points to each character, wanting to know the name, Amir wants to be able to answer. He finds it difficult to differentiate between Bert and Ernie, two characters who are always seen together. In looking for ways to associate the names with the characters, he notices that Bert has a much bigger head. He thinks, "Bert—big! Both words begin with B. That's how I'll remember."

Mrs. Rundle has allergies to dust, animals, weeds, and grasses. At her doctor's office, she was given samples of two allergy medications to try. One of the medications was to be taken in the morning because it can cause sleeplessness; the other was to be taken in the evening because it can be sedating. When she got home, Mrs. Rundle had forgotten the doctor's instructions. Because there were no directions on the sample packages, Mrs. Rundle had to call the doctor's office for clarification. She decided to make a conscious effort to remember which medication was which. She noted that the daytime medicine was blue, and she associated the color with the blue daytime sky.

Retrieval

Retrieval is the process of getting information from long-term memory into the conscious state of working memory. Most memory complaints center on the inability to bring information to mind on demand. In actuality, however, our ability to find a piece of information in our vast storehouse of memories and bring it to awareness is truly amazing and happens easily most of the time.

There are two ways you can retrieve information from long-term memory: recognition and recall.

Recognition is the perception of information that is presented to you as something or someone you already know. For example, you recognize the name of your friend's son when you hear her say it, but you could not come up with it on your own.

Recall is a self-initiated search of long-term memory for information you want. For example, you want to talk about your representative in Congress and need to search your memory bank for his name.

In most cases recognition is easier than recall. When you say, "I can't remember," you usually mean, "I can't recall." If you cannot recall the name of your representative in Congress, you may easily recognize it when you hear it. It may be hard to recall the name of a particular TV show, but you recognize it easily when you see it in the TV program section of your local newspaper.

Recall of information can be difficult because you must find one piece of information among the millions that are stored in long-term memory.

Sometimes recall of information is triggered by a cue. A **cue** is an event, thought, picture, word, sound, or something else that triggers the retrieval of information from long-term memory. For example, you may be able to recall the last name of your congressman when prompted with his first name. This triggering information, his first name, is a cue.

People often say, "I can't remember names, but I never

forget a face." We remember faces easily because they present themselves for **recognition**. Remembering names, on the other hand, involves **recall** of information from long-term memory, for which the face is only a **cue**.

When we are searching for a name or another piece of information, we can think of related facts, which may serve as cues and will often trigger the desired piece of information. For example, if you are having trouble recalling what course you took in summer school, you might think about where it was held, who was in the class with you, and other subjects you have taken in the past.

EXERCISE: *RECALL*

To answer the following questions, you are required to recall the information from long-term memory. If you find this task difficult, try to see if you can recognize the correct answers to the questions as they are asked again on page 23.

1. What is the capital city of Illinois?
2. Who played Dorothy in the movie *The Wizard of Oz*?
3. What is the name of the island in the Pacific Ocean that is famous for a photograph of U.S. Marines raising the American flag after a fierce battle with the Japanese?
4. Who was vice president of the United States in Richard Nixon's first administration?

See page 129 for answers.

4 Why We Forget

No one can remember everything. An essential part of the memory process is making decisions about what information is valuable to you and worth the effort to encode it. Is it really critical to spend energy encoding the name of a woman who occasionally teaches your exercise class when she is only an infrequent substitute? It might be better to choose to learn the names of your grandson's new wife and her parents.

Most people feel very frustrated and even embarrassed when they have to say, "I've forgotten." Before you blame a faulty memory, it's important to understand that there are some good reasons for not remembering.

1. **Some information never gets into the memory bank.** It gets only as far as sensory memory or working memory. Why? You didn't pay attention to it. You didn't really hear it. You didn't understand it. You didn't care enough to remember it. You got distracted by something else. You didn't need to remember it.

2. **Memories that do enter the memory bank may be overlaid with subsequent similar information that makes the original memory irretrievable.** People often describe their inadequacies in memory by saying, "I can't even remember what I ate for breakfast yesterday." If you eat similar types of break-

fast food day after day, you may forget what you ate on any particular morning, while the memory of the one time you ate octopus remains firm.

3. **Information for which you have few associations and little background knowledge is harder to remember.** For example, if you are just a beginner at the game of bridge, you will find it hard to remember any particular hand dealt during an evening of play, but a bridge expert can accurately recall all of the cards in a particularly meaningful hand.

4. **Some information may be remembered only when the proper cues are available, and those cues are not part of everyday life.** For example, you may think you've forgotten many of your eighth-grade classmates until you find an old photo or go to a class reunion.

5. **Who we are influences how we remember.** Many people assume that their own memories are a true picture of what really happened, and they are upset or confused by the conflicting recollections of others. Personal differences can affect encoding of information and can influence the way we remember; our background, knowledge, training, stance on life, age, gender, and prejudices all have an impact on the way we interpret events and commit them to memory. When two people remember things differently, they may argue over who is "forgetting." In reality, the difference in recollection may be due to the differing views and experiences of the people involved.

6. **Some pieces of remembered information may be assembled incorrectly.** Pieces of information may be recalled but misassembled. For example, you described to your cousin Emma a time when Uncle Bert fell out of a tree. She didn't remember the event, and you remarked that Aunt Rosemary didn't recall it, either. Several months later, you were amused

to hear Emma tell the same story and say she had heard it from Aunt Rosemary.

7. **Some memories fade away.** They are not readily available for all time. For example, if you studied a foreign language in high school, you may recall or recognize many of the vocabulary words you learned. Undoubtedly, however, you have no recollection of and no longer recognize many other words.

5   Let's Review

Let's review some of the terms used to describe the memory process.

Sensory memory: referring to the five senses through which all information enters the brain

Working memory: equated with conscious thought and holding the very small amount of information you can pay attention to at a given moment

Long-term memory: the accumulation of information that is not present in conscious thought but is stored for potential recollection

Encoding: learning and storing information

Retrieval: bringing information from long-term memory to conscious thought

Association: the connection between new information and what you already know

Recognition: perceiving information that is presented to you as something or someone you already know

Recall: a self-initiated search of long-term memory for information

Cue: the event, thought, picture, word, sound, or something else that triggers the retrieval of information from long-term memory

Here are those questions again. Are they easier this time?

EXERCISE: *RECOGNITION*

To answer the following questions, you are required to recognize the correct answers.

1. What is the capital city of Illinois?
   Chicago
   Peoria
   Springfield
   Champaign
2. Who played Dorothy in the movie *The Wizard of Oz?*
   Doris Day
   Judy Holliday
   Judy Garland
3. What is the name of the island in the Pacific Ocean that is famous for a photograph of U.S. Marines raising the American flag after a fierce battle with the Japanese?
   Oahu
   Iwo Jima
   Guam
4. Who was vice president of the United States in Richard Nixon's first administration?
   John Agnes
   Spiro Agnew
   Gerald Ford

See page 129 for answers.

EXERCISE: *UNDERSTANDING THE MEMORY PROCESS*

Complete the blanks in this scenario to test your understanding of the memory process. Use the words listed below.

    cue
    sensory memory
    association
    encoding
    long-term memory
    working memory
    retrieval

When you go to the library and notice a lot of colorful books on the "new books" shelf, the component of memory you are using is _____.
You read through the titles and think about whether they interest you. These conscious thoughts occur in the component of memory called _____.
Then you notice a book by a favorite author, John Grisham. You take down the book, notice how long it is, read the dust jacket, and decide you don't have time to read it this month. This process is called _____
_____.

The information about the book leaves your conscious thought and goes into the component of memory called

_____,

where it may be available for _____
at another time. When you get home, you notice another

of Grisham's books in your den. This favorite book serves
as a _____
to remind you of the book in the library. The connection
between the library book and your book at home is called
_____.

See page 129 for answers.

EXERCISE: *HOW MEMORY WORKS*

True/False. Circle the answer.

T F   1. Long-term memory refers to something that
          happened long ago.
T F   2. All information in conscious thought becomes
          part of your long-term memory.
T F   3. Sensory impressions may not register in con-
          scious thought.
T F   4. Associations are made both consciously and
          unconsciously.
T F   5. One piece of new information can be associ-
          ated with many different facts in your long-
          term memory.
T F   6. When you are presented with a name that
          you perceive as something you know, this
          form of retrieval is called recognition.
T F   7. Once information is encoded in long-term
          memory, it doesn't change.

See page 130 for answers.

II How Memory Changes as We Age

6   What Changes?
What Doesn't?

There are many myths about the inevitability of memory loss as people age. The truth is that the majority of older people will not face severe memory loss unless they have a serious illness such as Alzheimer's disease. Almost every older adult, however, is disturbed by memory changes that can be irritating and worrisome. It's very common to hear older people complain about forgetting names, forgetting what they read, misplacing things, or forgetting to do something important.

Researchers have extensively studied how memory changes with normal aging. Let's look at what they tell us about what happens to the components of the memory process over time. As we recall from chapter 2, the three components of the memory process are sensory memory, working memory, and long-term memory.

Sensory memory exhibits little change as people grow older. Older adults usually can register information through their senses in the same way they did when they were younger, unless there is significant vision or hearing loss. For example, Mrs. Bastien can scan the skeins of yarn in a knitting store to select the color she wants for an afghan. She can smell a melon to see whether it is ripe. Mr. Lopez can look through the selection of plants before choosing one for his garden. He can hear the birds in the back yard and feel happy.

Working memory—the amount of information you can pay attention to at any given moment—is much the same in older and younger people. Mrs. Bastien can think about how much yarn she needs and what color would suit her granddaughter. She can decide which melon to buy for the neighborhood potluck. Before making his selection, Mr. Lopez can think about the design of his garden and the amount of direct sunlight a plant requires. He can recognize a familiar bird call.

Long-term memory, information stored in the memory bank, is the component of memory most affected by age. The changes in long-term memory involve the ability to store and retrieve information efficiently.

As you recall from chapter 3, the process of storing information in long-term memory is called "encoding." The following common complaints demonstrate failures to encode information well enough:

- I can't keep track of where I put my glasses.
- I forget what people tell me.
- I hid some jewelry before I went on a trip, and I can't find it.

The second problem with long-term memory involves retrieval. You've already learned that retrieval can occur by recognition (the perception of information presented to you as something you already know) or by recall (a self-initiated search for information from long-term memory). The good news is that most people do not have problems with recognition: they say, "I know it when I see it" or "I know it when I hear it." In tests that measure knowledge and recognition of vocabulary words, older people do as well as or better than younger people. The retrieving of information on demand (recall), however, often becomes more difficult as we grow older.

Here are some examples of problems with recall:

- I forget names of people I should know.
- I can't remember the name of my medicine when someone asks me what I take.
- I can't remember how many teaspoons there are in a tablespoon.

Other problems could be failures of either encoding or recall, or both. For example:

- I can't remember what I read.
- I forgot an important appointment today.
- I heard a good joke, but I couldn't remember it well enough to tell.

So, why do encoding and recall become more difficult as we grow older? In chapters 7 and 8, we describe the changes in memory that come with age and affect our abilities to encode information and recall it on demand.

7 Problems with Encoding

It Becomes More Difficult to Pay Attention to More Than One Thing at a Time.

As you grow older, you may find it harder to attend to two competing activities, thoughts, or conversations. Keep in mind that the amount of information that can be held in working memory is quite limited, so what you are thinking of can be displaced even by your own new thought. Distractions such as a radio playing, someone talking, or a doorbell ringing may disrupt your concentration more now than they once did. The following examples present some common situations and potential solutions.

EXAMPLES

You are in the middle of a discussion at a party when you hear your name mentioned in a nearby conversation. This momentary distraction makes you lose track of what you are saying. You may feel embarrassed and blame your failing memory, but what has actually occurred is that one thought has displaced another in your working memory. This is a common experience, and you can simply say, "Where was I? I lost my train of thought."

You have several questions to ask your doctor. When she enters the exam room, you have them well in mind. Then she starts asking you about your health. You find that you no longer remember your questions. Remembering what you intend to ask your doctor at the same time that you are answering her questions involves a division of attention. If you go to your doctor with a written list of questions, you will not have to rely on your memory.

You are in the middle of baking bread when the thought of an old friend comes to mind. You daydream for a moment about the last time you were together. When you return to your baking, you realize you're not sure how many cups of flour you have added.

You are listening to the baseball game on the radio, eager to catch the score at the end of the inning. At the same time, you are sorting the mail. It seems reasonable to do these two things at once, but you suddenly realize the inning is over and you missed hearing the score. In the future, focus your attention on the game until the score is announced and then finish sorting the mail.

EXERCISE: *DIVIDED ATTENTION*

Can you add this column of figures while you continually repeat the names of the months of the year?

4
8
5
7
9

This exercise demonstrates how difficult it is to pay attention to two fairly simple tasks at one time.

ASSIGNMENT

During the next few days, notice if your attention is divided while you are trying to read the evening paper or listen to the news. Perhaps the phone rings, or you jump up to stir the soup. Maybe your spouse asks you a question. Think about whether these distractions affect your ability to remember what you are reading or listening to. Are you having a problem with your memory, or are you trying to attend to too many things at once?

It Takes Greater Effort to Learn Something New.

Too many people believe the myth that "you can't teach an old dog new tricks." However, unless there is impairment of the brain, people can continue to learn and remember throughout life. Researchers have found that older adults do need to exert greater effort to learn new information than they required in the past. The term "greater effort" means different things to different people. You will need to decide whether a task is worth the effort required. Read the following examples and see if you think the tasks are worth the effort.

EXAMPLE

Mariko may want to memorize the phone numbers of her four brothers and sisters and is willing to spend the necessary effort. She looks at the numbers for patterns and similarities. Some are easier than others to learn. She spends a total of an hour over the course of a week and learns them well. To keep them in her memory, she reviews them periodically. Suzanne may also have a goal of memorizing several phone numbers. After spending ten minutes trying, she thinks, "This isn't worth the effort. I can always look them up when I need them."

If you decide that it is important for you to remember some new information, you must focus your attention on the task and find some means of encoding the information. As you recall from chapter 3, encoding may include paying attention to something, analyzing it, associating it with something already known, and elaborating on the details.

EXAMPLES

Your city council has just enacted new regulations regarding the collection of recycled plastic. They will now accept certain plastic containers at curbside, while others are unacceptable. You regularly use, and would like to recycle, detergent, bleach, milk, cottage cheese, and yogurt containers. Because you keep forgetting which items are acceptable, you end up throwing them all in the trash. You decide that you want to easily remember which items to recycle without looking up the regulations or asking your neighbor each time.

The first step in learning this new information is giving your undivided attention to reading the information leaflet from the recycling center. You focus on the portion that describes what to do with plastics. The next step is thinking about how you can remember which of your commonly collected plastic items can go in the recycling bin. You note that the milk, bleach, and detergent containers are acceptable, whereas the cottage cheese and yogurt containers are not. After analyzing the situation, you realize that the three acceptable plastic items all contain liquids, whereas the others contain solids. Grouping these containers into other classifications, such as color, size, or shape, might also produce a solution to your problem.

You could easily have said, "It's too complicated for me. I can't remember all these distinctions." Instead you decided that it was important to learn and found a means of encoding the information.

Mrs. Kim has two friends named Gail and Gayle, one from her bridge club and the other from her neighborhood. She knows that they spell their names differently, but she can never remember which is which. The spelling of the name is important only when she sends her yearly holiday cards. Since she knows both friends well, she is concerned that she might misspell their names. She decides that she wants to be spared this quandary. She says to herself, "There must be a way to remember who is who." She calls a neighbor, who says that her friend from the neighborhood spells her name Gayle. She analyzes the spelling of the names and thinks about each person's characteristics. She realizes that GaYle is younger than Gail. "Y stands for younger!" she exclaims.

Mrs. Kim paid attention to the spelling of the names; she figured out a way to create an association between the spelling and the persons; she repeated the association aloud. All of these efforts resulted in deeply encoding the spelling of the names.

EXERCISE: *LEARNING NEW INFORMATION*

Here is some new information for you to learn and remember. Give it your undivided attention, and see how much effort it requires for you to answer the questions that follow the reading. The challenge is to find a way to remember the material, even if the particular subject does not interest you and it takes greater effort to remember than you thought it would.

Cognitive Behavioral Therapy (CBT) is a brief form of psychotherapy used in the treatment of mood problems, such as depression or anxiety. CBT helps people to

1. identify and correct inaccurate thoughts associated with depressed or anxious feelings,
2. engage more often in enjoyable activities, and
3. improve problem-solving skills.

The first step involves being aware of and correcting errors in thinking that are associated with problems in mood. For example, people with depression or anxiety often have distorted thoughts about themselves ("I am worthless" or "I can't do things as well as others"), their environments ("No one cares about me" or "My life is a mess"), or their futures ("I have nothing to look forward to" or "Something bad is going to happen to me").

In addition to thinking inaccurate thoughts, people with mood problems typically cut back on enjoyable activities because they think that such activities will not be worth the effort. For example, they may stop going to neighborhood gatherings or reading the newspaper. Unfortunately, this withdrawal usually results in a vicious cycle where depressed or anxious mood leads to less activity, which in turn results in further mood problems. The second step of CBT seeks to remedy this downward spiral by increasing rewarding activity.

The third step of CBT provides instruction and guidance in specific strategies for solving problems (for example, breaking problems down into small steps). If a person wanted to meet new people, perhaps the first step might be to look into volunteer opportunities.

Now, can you answer these questions about this new information?

1. Who could benefit from cognitive behavioral therapy?
2. What is an example of a distorted thought?
3. If a person is depressed, are they more or less likely to be active?
4. What is one strategy for solving problems?

See page 130 for answers.

8 Problems with Recall

It Is Increasingly Difficult to Access Familiar Names and Vocabulary Words on Demand.

Everyone knows the experience of being halted in midsentence when the desired word or name does not immediately spring to mind. The feeling of the word being on the tip of your tongue occurs more frequently as you age. The frustration of this experience can make you feel anxious, and this anxiety further blocks the recall process. You may have experienced something similar to Javier or Sukie in the following examples.

EXAMPLES

Javier began to tell a friend about the movie he saw last night, and he was astonished and embarrassed to discover that the title had escaped him. The more irritated he became, the less able he was to come up with the title. Instead of giving himself time and cues to retrieve the name of the movie from long-term memory, he found his attention focused on the frustration of forgetting.

Sukie started to tell a friend about the new bird feeder she had put up. "I saw a beautiful cardinal at the bird feeder on my . . . " At that moment the word "porch" escaped her, and she got flustered and said "the outside of my living room." This is a common occurrence that happens to everyone but is experienced more frequently as we grow older.

The next time you find yourself searching for a needed name or word, try to relax, take a deep breath, and see if you can access the information by thinking of related items. If you are still unable to retrieve that needed word, don't fret. It will undoubtedly come to you unbidden while you are thinking of something else.

It Takes Longer to Recall Information from Long-Term Memory.

Studies have shown that older adults take more time than younger people to recall needed information from long-term memory. When older adults are given increased time to complete a test, their performances are greatly improved. Keep this in mind when you are impatient with yourself because you don't recall something immediately. As in the following example, give yourself a little more time, and see if you can come up with the information you want.

EXAMPLE

Carol was talking to her daughter-in-law Inez on the telephone. Inez asked, "What did you do last night?" Carol hesitated and then responded, "Well, I guess, . . . nothing." Several seconds later, she exclaimed, "Oh, I remember! We went to see a movie. I just couldn't think of it for a minute." This information was clearly not forgotten; it just took Carol a little time to retrieve it from long-term memory.

Expertise and familiarity in a specific area often more than compensate for the slowing down of recall. For example, a seventy-year-old crossword-puzzle buff, who spends some time every day in this endeavor, may be able to recall words commonly needed in crossword puzzles as quickly as or more quickly than most younger people.

People Gain Knowledge and Wisdom with Age.

World knowledge, which is defined as a pool of information acquired over a lifetime from both educational and everyday experiences, accumulates with age. In tests that measure knowledge and vocabulary, older adults do as well as or better than younger people. The experiences of a long and rich life can produce a wisdom that young people can only hope to obtain. Memory and experience are the basis of wisdom. Although it takes greater effort to learn something new, older adults have the wisdom to determine what new information is important to them.

EXERCISE: *HOW MEMORY CHANGES*

True / False. Circle the answer.

T   F   1. There is no escaping significant memory loss as you grow older.

T   F   2. If you have always been able to do several things at once, age won't affect this ability.

T   F   3. Sensory and working memory show little change as people grow older.

T   F   4. Older adults take longer to recall information from long-term memory.

T   F   5. Older adults find recognition more difficult than recall.

T   F   6. One way to access well-known information when you can't recall it is to provide yourself with cues by thinking of related items.

See page 130 for answers.

III Factors That Affect Memory

9 You and Your Memory: A Self-inventory

Pauline recently moved from Collinsville, Illinois, her lifelong hometown, to an apartment building near her son's home in Chicago. She had mixed feelings about moving. In Collinsville she had many friends and was active in volunteer work at the school. She regularly attended an exercise class and always went out for lunch after church with the same group of people. After her husband died, however, she decided it would be best to move nearer to her son and his family. The move was stressful because she had to reduce the belongings of a family home to fit the space of a two-bedroom apartment. She spent many weeks making decisions about what to take and how to get rid of unwanted items. By the time she arrived in her new apartment, she was too exhausted to organize things well. She missed her friends at home and found it hard to meet new people and get involved in activities. She found herself feeling sad and somewhat hopeless about creating a satisfying new life in Chicago.

For the first time, Pauline began to question her memory. She couldn't find her address book in her new apartment. She got lost driving back from the library. She fell asleep after putting some potatoes on to boil and woke up to the smell of a burned pan. She said to herself, "What is happening to me?

Maybe I'm getting Alzheimer's disease."

Pauline made an appointment with a geriatrician and expressed her fears about her memory. Dr. Sloan reviewed her recent history and did some tests. He assured Pauline that she didn't have Alzheimer's, explaining that many factors in her recent experience could temporarily affect her memory.

Certain factors can affect memory for people of all ages. The effect of these factors is likely to be greater as we age because older people often experience more of these negative influences at one time. The following factors commonly affect memory:

Attitude and effort
    Problems with paying attention
    Negative expectations
    Inactivity
    Lack of organization in daily life
Problems with mood
    Depression
    Loss and grief
    Anxiety
    Stress
Health issues
    Physical illnesses
    Medications
    Vision and hearing problems
    Fatigue
    Alcohol
    Poor nutrition

As you read through the next three chapters, think about which of these factors might be affecting your memory. If you are aware of the possible causes of memory problems, you are more likely to find solutions.

10 Take a Look at Your Effort and Attitude

The first step in assessing your memory is to determine whether there is anything about your attitude or effort that might be getting in the way of your memory. Take a look at the four factors discussed in this chapter (problems with attention, negative expectations, inactivity, lack of organization). Are any of them creating problems for you? Do you recognize yourself in any of the examples?

Problems with Attention

Inadequate Attention

In the discussion of encoding in chapter 3, we emphasized the importance of focusing attention on what you want to remember. If you really want to remember something, paying adequate attention is the first step. In the following examples, inadequate attention affected the encoding of new information.

EXAMPLES

A new resident of Brad's apartment building, Lia Blair, meets him at the mailboxes and introduces herself. He greets her by name and begins a friendly conversation. When they are joined by another resident a few minutes later, Brad discovers that he has no recollection of Lia's name.

Ramona bought some expensive concert tickets and made a mental note to take them out of her purse when she got home and put them in a special place so she could easily find them later. The next morning, as she got in her car to leave for work, she realized she hadn't put the tickets safely away, nor could she find the tickets in her purse. She went back to her apartment and found them on the kitchen table. She was relieved to know that the tickets weren't lost, but she couldn't understand why she had no recollection of having put them on the table.

Both of these examples illustrate problems in encoding. Brad heard and spoke Lia Blair's name but didn't encode the information into long-term memory for recollection. Ramona absentmindedly took the tickets from her purse and placed them on the table. She had not paid adequate attention to what she was doing.

Paying adequate attention to details can eliminate some instances of forgetting. Ask yourself, "When is it really important for me to pay attention?" At these times, put some effort into focusing your awareness on the task or information at hand.

Distractions

Another potential problem with attention is the presence of distractions. Because the amount of information that can be held in your working memory is quite limited, any sound, sight, or thought may distract you and displace what is currently in your working memory. You are certain to have had one or more of the following experiences.

EXAMPLES

You go into the kitchen to get the scissors and forget what you went for. Perhaps, on your way, you wondered whether the mail had come. This new thought replaced the thought of the scissors you needed from the kitchen.

You may leave your umbrella in the doctor's office because you are thinking about getting your prescription filled before the drugstore closes.

You're driving to a movie with a friend. Her conversation draws your attention from noticing exactly where you are, and you forget to get into the left-turn lane until it's too late.

These experiences are familiar to people of all ages, but older adults do find it more difficult to pay attention to more than one thing at a time. Rather than thinking that you can do nothing about these frustrating experiences, try to recognize the limitations of working memory and cut out distractions when possible. It is especially important to give your undivided attention to situations that could be potentially dangerous, such as driving, cooking, and taking medications. For example, when driving in an unfamiliar place, you might want to ask your passenger to stop talking until you arrive.

EXERCISE: *DISTRACTIONS*

Below are two short stories. Read the first one in a quiet room, and then read the second one with some competition for your attention, such as the TV or radio.

First Story
A grandmother and grandfather and their two preschool grandchildren went for a drive in their red van on a rainy day. They passed a fruit stand and decided to turn back to buy some sweet cherries and squash. They drove to a diner and had a turkey dinner with corn and biscuits. They returned home on a gravel road, where they were chased by a barking dog.

Second Story
A lifeguard at a rocky beach came to work on his silver motorcycle. He changed from blue jeans to a green bathing suit and put his whistle around his neck. He hollered at three teen-agers, who were out too far, to come closer to shore. At sunset, his blond girlfriend brought him a hot dog, a Coke, and some potato chips.

Did you notice differences in your ability to remember the details in these two stories?

Negative Expectations

Compared to younger people, older adults are more pessimistic about their ability to remember. Older people often say, "I just can't remember anything anymore," whereas younger people blame forgetting on a lack of effort. When you expect that you are going to fail at something, that expectation is likely to increase the possibility of failure. Negative attitudes about memory often cause older people to

- put less effort into remembering
- avoid tasks that require memory
- feel anxious when their memories are tested in daily life

EXAMPLE

Agnes Martin attended a volunteer appreciation banquet. Although she recognized many faces, she felt embarrassed and anxious when she could not address people by name. She thought, "I can't remember names anymore!" Since that time she has avoided attending gatherings when she doesn't know everyone extremely well. Although her son-in-law gave her a book on how to remember names, she is sure that those techniques are not useful for someone of her age.

When you are faced with a task of memory, do you find yourself saying, "I'll never be able to do this. What's the use of trying?" Sometimes we give ourselves negative messages without being aware of it. Be conscious of your self-defeating thoughts about your ability to remember. Substitute this thought: "I'm not sure this will work, but I'll give it a good try."

Inactivity

We frequently read that mental, social, and physical activity are good for the mind and body. As you read this section, think about whether increased activity might benefit your memory. Examine your attitude and effort to see whether your outlook is affecting your level of activity.

Lack of Mental Stimulation

The old adage "Use it or lose it" is often applied to memory functioning. Keeping mentally active and using memory skills may enhance your ability to remember. Here are some examples of mental stimulation:

- attending an adult education class
- participating in a discussion group
- doing crossword puzzles
- playing bridge, chess, or Trivial Pursuit
- answering *Jeopardy* or other quiz show questions
- learning to use a computer
- reading a challenging book
- using newly learned memory techniques

EXAMPLE

Karen has always had a great interest in current events. Although she reads the newspaper daily, she has lately found it difficult to retain the information needed to formulate her position on issues. Rather than give up, she joins the current events discussion group in her senior apartment building. She enjoys the lively discussions and finds that her memory for issues is reinforced by preparing for the group and hearing the opinions of others.

Lack of Social Interaction

Many people agree that social involvement is a major factor in maintaining or improving mental capacities. When days are uncommitted and unstructured, there is less incentive to focus and organize your thoughts and less need to remember.

In social contact you have the opportunity to talk about the events of your life, which reinforces the memory of what you have done and learned.

EXAMPLES

You receive a letter from your daughter telling you that your granddaughter is running for class president. When your daughter calls later in the week and says, "Jenny won!" you have no idea what she is talking about. Before you assume that your memory is failing, consider the fact that you saw very few people over the week and told no one about the news. If you tell a friend about any new information you receive, you encode it more deeply and greatly increase your chances of remembering it.

Mr. Polanski is eighty-eight years old and lives alone with no relatives nearby. He suffers from severe arthritis and heart problems. He is uncomfortable and fearful when away from home. His neighbor brings in his mail each day and notices that Mr. Polanski is becoming more forgetful. He rarely knows what day it is and has forgotten his last two doctors' appointments. When he finally sees the doctor, Mr. Polanski has an ulcer on his foot that needs attention. The doctor orders a visiting nurse and a home health aide three times a week to provide personal care and homemaking services. After a few weeks, Mr. Polanski's neighbor notices that he seems more alert and always remembers what day it is, since he looks forward to the aide coming on Monday, Wednesday, and Friday. The interaction with the aide has improved his memory for recent events as they share conversations about daily living and current events.

Lack of Physical Activity

Recent research studies have shown that both sick and healthy older people who exercise regularly are more likely to maintain mental functioning ability. In other words, routine exercise programs are good for both the body and the mind. In one study, however, participants who exercised for a while and then stopped lost the benefits they had gained.

EXAMPLE

Zella has been afraid of falling on the ice during a severe winter in Minnesota and has hardly left the house. She can't remember much about what happened yesterday or the day before. She's afraid that her memory is failing along with her health. Friends have been trying to get her to go to an exercise class, but she just hasn't felt like it. One day she finally gives in and goes to senior aerobics. She finds it difficult for the first couple of weeks, but since she has paid for an eight-week class, she sticks with it. After about a month, Zella notices that she has more energy and that her mind seems a bit sharper. She reads an article in the paper about the relationship between physical exercise and mental functioning. She thanks her friend and says, "Maybe this class will be good for my mind as well as my body."

Lack of Organization in Daily Life

Many instances of forgetting and losing things can be traced to a disorganized lifestyle. When you don't have a systematic way to keep track of your appointments, return things to their correct places in your home, pay bills, or store important papers in a safe place, you are more likely to be forgetful. Many people have developed a lifelong habit of being organized, while others are disorganized and have never been bothered by it. If you think that some of your instances of forgetting are due to a lack of organization, you may want to develop some new organizational habits. It does take effort to make changes, but organization saves effort in the long run.

EXAMPLES

Phyllis complained, "I always write things down. I know about keeping lists, but then I can't find the lists." At a memory course at her recreation center, she heard other participants describe the same situation. The teacher advised them to keep all lists of things to buy or do in one convenient place. Phyllis realized she had been making lists on odd scraps of paper and leaving them all over the house. She remedied the situation by keeping a notebook for lists on her kitchen table.

You notice that your credit card bill is unusually large. You're positive that you paid last month's bill, but when you look in the checkbook there is no record of payment. You search for the bill in all the likely places with no success. After you've called the credit card company to complain, you discover last month's bill in a book you're reading. No wonder you forgot to pay it! Most people can't keep track of household finances without some organized system. When your bills are scattered throughout the house and you have no regular schedule for paying them, it's very easy to neglect one.

ASSIGNMENT

Choose **one** area of your life in which you think getting organized will help you remember:

_____ Keeping track of my purse / keys / glasses / umbrella /_____

_____ Remembering when I last gave to my favorite charity

_____ Sending birthday cards to family and friends on time

_____ Paying my bills when they're due

_____ Keeping track of the scissors / tape / pencil sharpener / wrapping paper /_____

_____ Putting gas in the car before it's nearly empty

_____ Remembering to take the garbage out

_____ Your choice _____

Now that you have chosen one, think of a way to organize this area of your life so you will remember. For example, you might put up a hook where you will **always** hang your keys.

The problem:

_____

_____

_____

Your solution:

_____

_____

_____

The results:

_____

_____

_____

After you have accomplished this goal, why not choose another?

The problem:

_____

_____

_____

Your solution:

_____

_____

_____

The results:

_____

_____

_____

11 Could Your Mood Be the Problem?

You may be surprised to learn that your mood can affect your memory. If you are experiencing depression, grief, anxiety, or stress, you may not recognize the symptoms or realize that these conditions can create problems with memory. We hope this chapter and its examples will help you evaluate your mood and its effect on your memory.

Depression

Many people believe that depression is a normal part of aging, but depression is not normal. It is an illness—a very treatable illness. We know that memory problems often accompany depression, but if the depression is treated, the memory problems improve. Some symptoms of depression are

- appetite change (decrease in appetite is most common)
- sleep disturbance
- fatigue
- anxiety, fearfulness, excessive worrying
- feelings of hopelessness or helplessness
- decreased concentration, difficulty with memory
- difficulty making decisions

- restlessness, pacing
- irritability
- feeling that life is not worth living
- feeling that nothing gives you pleasure
- feeling sick or tired all the time
- sad mood
- suicidal thoughts

How does depression affect memory?

Motivation: When you are depressed you don't care about remembering your new neighbor's name, the time of your exercise class, or who's running for city council. None of these things seems important.

Concentration: Even if you want to remember how to fill out your Medicare form, depression can make you feel foggy and unable to focus on the task.

Perception: If you are depressed you may view a few instances of forgetting as a sign that you can't remember anything at all.

EXAMPLE

Ed has experienced bouts of depression for several years. His friends and family noticed that, when he was feeling depressed, he forgot appointments, confused the names of his grandchildren, and couldn't remember what happened the day before. The first few times this occurred, his family wondered if he were getting Alzheimer's disease. The family encouraged Ed to see his physician. After a full evaluation Dr. Garcia concluded that Ed's memory problems might improve if his depression were treated by a combination of medication and counseling. He also suggested that, until Ed's depression improved, he should use as many memory aids as possible.

Loss and Grief

When you have experienced a significant loss, you are often overwhelmed with feelings of pain and sadness. It is difficult to focus on anything outside yourself, and your ability to concentrate is diminished. Memory problems frequently accompany grief and will lessen over time unless the mourner becomes severely depressed.

When we talk about loss and grief, most people think primarily of death. In fact, a feeling of loss may accompany many different experiences, including moving, major surgery, retirement of yourself or your spouse, vision or hearing impairment, illness of a friend or family member, changes in financial circumstances, death of a pet, marriage of a child or friend, and changes in your own health. When two or more of these experiences occur at once, the effect is greatly increased.

EXAMPLES

Harry had been ready to retire for several years when the day finally arrived. He looked forward to sleeping late, having no boss to answer to, and spending time in his basement workshop. He was surprised to discover, however, that he often felt sad and at loose ends. He also noticed that he was forgetting things. With his wife's encouragement, he volunteered to deliver Meals on Wheels to shut-ins and began a drawing class. As he felt more useful, his sadness diminished, along with much of his forgetfulness. Even a change you choose to make can be accompanied by a feeling of loss.

Ken had been dating Josephine for a year and a half. He thought things were going well and planned on a future with her. After the holidays, Josephine told him that she hadn't been happy in their relationship for a while and that she wanted to stop seeing him. Ken initially was very angry and told himself he was better off without her. As days passed, he found himself tearful and overwhelmed. He couldn't pay attention to his work and forgot his grandson's birthday party. He suddenly felt like his mind was old and decrepit. He wondered if he was losing his memory, but he didn't know what to do about it. After several months passed, he realized that he was feeling better and that his memory was better, too. With the lessening of Ken's grief, his memory returned to normal.

Anxiety

Anxiety is characterized as inner distress accompanied by physical symptoms and vague fears. Many people who are highly anxious are unable to focus on anything outside of themselves. Their minds are so filled with worries that they cannot pay attention to external happenings, and their memory failures affect their daily functioning.

Some symptoms of anxiety are

- nervousness, worry, or fear
- apprehension or a sense of imminent doom
- panic spells
- difficulty concentrating
- insomnia
- fear of potential physical illnesses
- heart pounding or racing
- upset stomach or diarrhea
- sweating
- dizziness or light-headedness
- restlessness or jumpiness
- irritability

EXAMPLE

Eva describes herself as someone who has always been a worrier, but it has gotten worse as she has grown older. She worries about her unmarried son, her granddaughter's thumb-sucking, her own high blood pressure, and her arthritis, which could affect her ability to take care of her home. She has butterflies in her stomach, she doesn't sleep well, she spends most of the day worrying, and she is unable to remember things very well.

When she is in the clinic to get a blood pressure reading, Eva mentions her anxiety to the nurse, who suggests that she should discuss it with the doctor. Dr. Persky recommends a cognitive therapy group for people who are anxious or depressed, where Eva might learn new ways of dealing with her anxiety and benefit from the group support. In the group, Eva recognizes that she has no control over her son's unmarried state and her granddaughter's thumb-sucking. She vows to try to take them off her worry list. The group helps her consider some options for the future in case she is unable to take care of her home. Eva knows that she will continue to be a worrier; however, when she realized the uselessness of worrying about those things that she cannot control and began to make plans for her future, some of her symptoms of anxiety were alleviated, including her memory problems. As she worried less, she found she could concentrate and remember better.

Stress

When you are feeling stressed, anxious, pressured, or rushed, it is often impossible to

- pay adequate attention to learning new information
- concentrate on the details you want to recall
- relax long enough to let a memory surface

You are more likely to forget things when you are under major stress—due to factors such as moving, illness, loss, your own retirement, or the retirement of your spouse—or even when you are under minor stress caused by experiences such as being late to an appointment, misplacing your house keys, preparing for company, or seeing your doctor. It is important to realize that you may forget more frequently at times like these and that your memory usually improves as the stress is reduced. When you add worry about forgetting to other stresses, you often increase forgetfulness.

EXAMPLE

You have been extremely busy all week getting ready for a visit from your son and his family, who live in California. The sink becomes clogged, and the plumber is available only during the time when you are picking up the family from the airport. You ask your neighbor if you can give her a house key when you leave for the airport, so she can let the plumber in. To your horror, you forget to leave the key. Because you were stressed, overloaded, and rushing, you forgot to do what you wanted to do most. In a case like this, it's best to leave the key the moment you think of it.

---

12 Ask Your Doctor about Health Issues

EXAMPLE

Ellen Singer's son is very concerned about her forgetfulness. He continually tells her that she should try harder and feels that she should learn some new memory techniques. He reads about a memory course in the local newspaper and insists that his mother enroll in the course, although she is not enthusiastic. He calls the instructor to enroll her in the class and describes her problems. She repeats herself frequently and sometimes forgets that he has called. She is having trouble balancing her checkbook and has dropped out of her card-playing group. As he paints the picture of his mother's memory problems and expresses his conviction that she could remember if she really tried, the instructor wonders whether Mrs. Singer's memory problems may be related to a health issue. She suggests to the son that he should go with his mother to her next medical appointment and discuss his concerns with her doctor.

Physical health and mental functioning are very closely linked. Factors such as physical illnesses, medications, vision and hearing problems, fatigue, alcohol, and nutrition may require consultation with a health care provider. Ask your doctor whether your memory changes may be related to a health problem or medication.

Some Physical Illnesses

Even though most older people do not develop severe memory loss, memory problems can be a sign that the body is not functioning properly. Some physical illnesses can aggravate an already existing mild memory problem, or they can cause memory changes in a person who has previously exhibited no memory loss.

Minor conditions, such as infection, fever, dehydration, and thyroid problems, can cause temporary changes in memory that improve when the condition is treated.

On the other hand, some types of diseases or injuries that cause damage to the brain may not be reversible. Alzheimer's disease is the major cause of irreversible memory loss (see the Appendix). Strokes and traumatic injury to the head often cause memory problems that show improvement in the months after the trauma but frequently leave some irreversible changes. Parkinson's disease can also affect memory and other cognitive functions. Some less common diseases that cause memory problems are Creutzfeldt-Jakob disease, normal pressure hydrocephalus, Pick's disease, Lewy body disease, and Huntington's disease.

If you are concerned about your memory and want to rule out a physical cause, the first step is to see your family doctor, who is familiar with your medical history. Some physicians, however, receive little training in assessing the mental status of older people. Therefore, it may be worthwhile to consult a physician with specific training in geriatrics or neurology, who has the diagnostic skills to distinguish among a wide assortment of possible causes of memory loss. A medical assessment often includes

- a social and medical history taken from both the patient and a relative or friend
- a thorough physical examination
- a neuropsychological exam, which is a series of tests that provide information about the thought processes
- blood tests, which are used to detect thyroid, kidney, and liver malfunctions; certain nutritional deficiencies, such as pernicious anemia or vitamin B_{12} deficiency; infections; and metabolic and chemical imbalances
- urinalysis, which is used to detect infections

Other possible tests that may be indicated include

- CT scan (computerized axial tomogram): a special x-ray of the brain
- MRI (magnetic resonance imaging): a procedure that painlessly scans the brain and other body parts using no radiation
- EEG (electroencephalogram): a measurement of electrical activity (brain waves) in the brain
- lumbar puncture (spinal tap): an analysis of spinal fluid that can detect malignancies, neurosyphilis, and certain infections
- PET scan (positron emission tomogram): a nuclear medicine scan of the brain

In the following example, the sudden change in Mrs. Vincenti's cognitive status indicates a physical cause.

EXAMPLE

When Cathy, the housecleaner, arrived at Mrs. Vincenti's apartment for her weekly visit, she found Mrs. Vincenti in bed and quite confused. When Cathy asked her if she had had breakfast, Mrs. Vincenti said she wasn't sure. Also, she could not remember Cathy's name or exactly why Cathy was there. Since Mrs. Vincenti had never been so confused in the past, Cathy consulted with a neighbor, who agreed that Mrs. Vincenti should go to the emergency room. The physicians at the hospital discovered that she had a serious urinary tract infection and admitted her to the hospital. When Mrs. Vincenti's infection cleared up, her confusion disappeared, and she returned home feeling mentally and physically well.

Some Medications

Prescription and over-the-counter medications can affect your memory because they can slow your thinking and make you feel drowsy or foggy. They can diminish your attention or concentration, making it harder to register information in your working memory.

Most, but not all, of the time, memory is affected within days after starting a new medication or increasing the dose. Sometimes the change is noticed by the person taking the medication, and sometimes the change is more noticeable to other people. A memory problem due to medication is seldom permanent, however. In fact, the problem may go away on its own as you continue to take the medicine and your body adjusts to it. If the problem doesn't go away, talk with your doctors to find out whether there are other medications you can take instead.

No one can tell who will have a memory problem from a medication, and it can happen to anyone. Some things, however, make a person more likely to have memory problems with medications:

- low weight
- older age
- a sudden change in health
- taking other medications
- taking more (or less) of a medication than you are supposed to
- taking a medication in combination with alcohol
- a medical condition like Alzheimer's disease that is already affecting memory
- some kinds of liver disease
- kidney disease

Although some medications affect memory and attention more than others do, the same medications don't cause the same problems in everyone. Medications that have a higher risk of memory problems include

- prescription sleeping or anxiety medications
  Ambien (zolpidem)
  Ativan (lorazepam)
  Halcion (triazolam)
  Restoril (temazepam)
  Sonata (zaleplon)
  Valium (diazepam)
  Xanax (alprazolam)
- muscle relaxants
  Lioresal (baclofen)

Flexeril (cyclobenzaprine)
Skelaxin (metaxalone)
Soma (carisoprodol)
Neurontin (gabapentin)
- some allergy or cold medicines
Benadryl (diphenhydramine)
Chlor-Trimeton (chlorpheniramine)
- some pain medications
MS Contin and other brands of morphine
Duragesic or Actiq (fentanyl)
hydrocodone (found in Vicodin and other brands)
Oxycontin and other brands of oxycodone

Memory problems can happen at any time during treatment, but they happen more often when getting started or when increasing the dose.

Medications are only one of many causes of memory problems. If you think you are having a memory problem from a medication, you should talk to your doctor or pharmacist. **Never stop taking or reduce your medications on your own.** Together, you and your doctor can decide whether your memory problem may be due to the medication and what to do about it.

When it comes to side effects of medicines, prevention is key. You can be a partner in preventing memory problems due to medications by

- keeping a list of medications and showing it to your doctors and pharmacists before you start or change the dose of a medicine
- working with your doctors to try to stop medications you may no longer need

- not drinking alcohol if you think your memory might be affected by your medications
- talking with your doctors or pharmacists about scheduling the taking of your medications to lessen their effect on your memory
- telling your doctors and pharmacists if you think your memory is affected by a medicine, so they can try to prevent this problem from happening again with the same or similar medications

(This section on medications was written by Tami Remington, Pharm.D., Clinical Assistant Professor, University of Michigan, Ann Arbor.)

EXAMPLE

Jerome has been feeling tired and foggy, and he is forgetting more than he used to. His daughter suggests that he see his family doctor for consultation. Dr. Brown takes a complete history, including a review of medications. She discovers that Jerome has begun to take over-the-counter antihistamines to control his seasonal allergies, along with the sleeping pills that she had prescribed at the last visit. Dr. Brown recognizes that the combination of the two drugs may be causing Jerome's fatigue and memory problems. She prescribes a shorter-acting sleeping pill, so that this medication will be out of Jerome's system during the daytime. She also substitutes a nonsedating allergy medication for the antihistamine. Jerome finds that, over time, his memory improves with this combination of medications.

Vision and Hearing Problems

An older person with vision or hearing problems often blames his memory if he can't recall information or experiences. In fact, the problem may not be in the memory at all. When you can't see or hear clearly, the information will not be encoded correctly. It is important to admit when you can't hear adequately and ask others to speak up. If you are unable to read printed material, ask for a large-print copy or ask someone to read it to you. Frequent vision and auditory tests are necessary to ensure that you're getting the aids you need. Vision and hearing abilities can change dramatically, and new technology may compensate for losses.

EXAMPLES

Your neighbor suggests that you call a Realtor whose name is Abbott. When you call the realty company, you ask for Mr. Babcock. The problem here may not be your memory; your neighbor may have mumbled, or you may have trouble hearing. If you want to remember something correctly, ask the person to repeat it, spell it, or even write it down.

At the doctor's office, the receptionist gives you an insurance form to complete at home. "Just sign in these three places, and mail it off," she says, pointing to three blanks. When you get home, you are confused by all the blank spaces and say, "I've already forgotten what she told me." The problem may not be in your memory. You may not have seen the spaces she pointed to. Next time, ask her to mark the spaces with a red X.

Fatigue

Fatigue affects your ability to concentrate and slows down the recall process. You are more likely to have trouble learning new information when you're tired. If you can figure out which times of the day you are most alert, you can do tasks that involve new learning at those times.

EXAMPLES

You usually read at bedtime because it puts you to sleep. However, you can't keep the characters straight in the book you're reading, and this frustrates you. You might try reading this book when you are more alert. If you want to read before dozing off, read something you don't care about remembering.

You have just finished the third lecture of a six-week series on health problems. You were especially looking forward to last week's lecture on diabetes because your husband has diabetes in his family. You realize, however, that you remember little of the material because you were especially tired that day. For the next lecture, you resolve to be rested and ready to take notes.

Alcohol

Alcohol can affect your memory in two different ways. First, many people find that they are less able to tolerate alcohol as they grow older; two drinks may have been tolerated well in the past but are now too much. The effects of alcohol are more dependent on the amount consumed during one drinking occasion than on how often a person takes a drink. As far as memory is concerned, there is a greater effect on the brain if you have four drinks in one night than if you have one drink on each of four nights. Second, long-term abuse of alcohol can cause irreversible memory loss.

In addition to the direct effects of alcohol on memory, alcohol consumption can cause or worsen other factors that affect your memory:

- Depression: Alcohol acts as a depressant on the central nervous system.
- Decreased nutritional status: Alcohol provides calories without nutritional content. Some people who drink excessively fail to eat an adequate diet.

Poor Nutrition

There is still a great deal to be learned about how nutrition affects memory, but we know that a well-balanced diet contributes to overall health. Some older people eat a limited range of foods, such as toast and canned soup, a diet that can lead to a deficiency of needed nutrients. Fresh fruits and vegetables, whole-grain cereals and breads, and low-fat dairy foods or meat should be eaten daily. Small, frequent meals can be easier to prepare than traditional, larger meals and may result in healthier eating habits and an adequate intake of calories. Maintaining the appropriate body weight for height and age is especially important. Being either underweight or overweight can be unhealthy.

The use of a normal-dosage multivitamin supplement is safe and appropriate if the reasons for an inadequate diet are not easily remedied. Megadoses of vitamins or minerals are not safe and should not be taken unless prescribed by a health care provider.

Older adults have increased sensitivity to caffeine, nicotine, and alcohol, all of which should be used in moderation or avoided altogether.

Community nutrition programs can help older adults maintain healthy eating habits. Eating with others is an important part of mealtime for many people. Many cities and towns have programs for seniors, offering meals and fellowship in communal settings. Outreach programs can help older adults shop for food, and homemaker services can help prepare meals in the home. For those who are homebound, some programs, such as Meals on Wheels, deliver meals to older adults.

(This section on nutrition was written by Kate Jones Share, M.S., Clinical Nutritionist, Ann Arbor, Michigan.)

13 Let's Review Again

Now that we've explained how different factors affect memory, think about which factors might be affecting you.

	Never	Some-times	Always
1. Problems with attention	_____	_____	_____
2. Negative expectations	_____	_____	_____
3. Inactivity	_____	_____	_____
4. Lack of organization	_____	_____	_____
5. Depression	_____	_____	_____
6. Loss and grief	_____	_____	_____
7. Anxiety	_____	_____	_____
8. Stress	_____	_____	_____
9. Physical illness	_____	_____	_____
10. Medication	_____	_____	_____
11. Vision problems	_____	_____	_____
12. Hearing problems	_____	_____	_____

13. Fatigue   _____ _____ _____
14. Alcohol   _____ _____ _____
15. Nutrition   _____ _____ _____

You may wish to go back now and reread the information in earlier chapters about the factors that are affecting you. Addressing some of these factors may require you to see a physician, counselor, or other professional for treatment. For other factors you may find ways to make changes in your environment or lifestyle to address the problem.

EXERCISE: *FACTORS THAT AFFECT MEMORY*

True / False. Circle the answer.

T F   1. Problems with vision or hearing can affect your memory.
T F   2. Memory is not affected by emotion.
T F   3. Poor memory is often due to lack of attention.
T F   4. Negative expectations have no effect on memory performance.
T F   5. Lack of concentration can be a symptom of anxiety or depression.
T F   6. Problems with your health can cause increased forgetting.
T F   7. Medications affect everyone the same way.
T F   8. Even if you're looking forward to moving to a new place, you may notice some memory problems after you move.

T   F   9. Once your memory begins to get worse, it
                will never improve.
T   F   10. Increasing activity, through mental stimula-
                tion, social interaction, or physical exercise,
                may benefit memory.

See page 131 for answers.

IV Techniques for Improving Your Memory

14 It's Time to Explore Strategies

So far we have learned about how memory works and about how memory changes with normal aging. We hope you have identified any factors in your life that may be affecting your memory. Now we are ready to explore strategies and techniques that can make a difference in your ability to remember.

Once you have determined that you want to improve your memory in a particular area, you can select strategies for change. In this chapter we introduce sixteen techniques for improving your memory. In the chapters that follow we describe these techniques and how to use them.

Some techniques improve the way you encode information so you can retrieve it more easily:

- association
- visualization
- active observation
- elaboration

Some techniques involve cues in your environment, such as notes, lists, signs, or buzzers:

- written reminders
- auditory reminders
- environmental change

One technique is extremely useful for remembering whether you did what you meant to do:

- self-instruction

Five techniques help when you have several items to remember:

- story method
- chunking
- first-letter cues
- create a word
- categorization

Some techniques are helpful in retrieving information that you know well but can't quite bring to mind:

- cue yourself
- alphabet search
- review in advance

Some of these techniques will be familiar; others will seem strange. It is difficult to know which ones will be useful for you without trying them several times. Look for chances to experiment.

It can be fun and rewarding to figure out a way to remember and then to succeed. We believe that there's a tool for remembering almost anything. In some cases, however, you may decide that the effort needed is not worth the benefit gained. Recognize that the choice is yours to make.

Here's the best way to use these memory improvement techniques:

1. Choose something specific that you want to remember.
2. Review the possible techniques and select one.
3. Try the technique. (If it works, congratulations!)
4. If your chosen technique does not work, try something else.
5. Don't feel defeated if some things are particularly hard to remember. Ask yourself whether it really matters anyway.

15 Improving Your Ability to Encode

Although there are many techniques for remembering specific kinds of information, there are four strategies you can use whenever you want to encode almost any kind of new information securely so that it is available for retrieval.

People who have excellent memories use these strategies on a daily basis. It takes thought and practice, but if you can incorporate these strategies into everyday life, you will have a better memory. All of the examples in this chapter illustrate strategies for encoding information more securely. The exercises give you a chance to practice these strategies.

Association: Associate What You Want to Remember with What You Already Know.

Association is the process of forming mental connections between what you want to remember and what you already know. Although many associations are made automatically, the conscious creation of an association is an excellent strategy for encoding new information. Once you make an association, repeating it several times either in your head or aloud will help you remember.

This technique can be used to remember such things as

- the name of your new neighbor
- the street where your friend lives
- the title of a movie you want to recommend
- whether to turn right or left to get to the restaurant
- the number of the bus to your friend's house

EXAMPLES

Beth: I had a new neighbor whose name was Marsha. For some reason I had a hard time remembering her name. I had learned about association in a memory course and decided to try it. After looking carefully at Marsha, I noticed she had white, fluffy hair. I decided that I could remember her name by associating "Marsha" with "marshmallow." Each time I saw her, I associated her hair with a big marshmallow and said to myself, "Marshmallow Marsha."

Leroy: I could never remember whether my gas tank is on the right or left side of the car. Each time I went to fill up, I had to think about which way to approach the gas pumps, and I felt aggravated. I decided to consciously find an association that would register the information once and for all. I first noted that my gas cap is on the right side. What could I associate with "right"? This was easier than I thought—I have a red car! I associated the "r" in red with the "r" in right. Now when I go to the gas station, I say, "In this red car, the gas cap is on the right." Problem solved!

(You may be saying to yourself, "Sure—he happens to have a red car with the gas tank on the right. What about my car that is black and the gas tank is on the right?" In this case, you may need to go beyond the obvious. You may notice that both "black" and "right" have five letters. Again, problem solved! However, if you can't find an association between your car and its gas tank, you need a different strategy. How about repeating "Right is right" or "Left is logical"? That should do the trick.)

EXERCISE: *ASSOCIATION*

Create an association between the following items of new information and something you already know.

1. You must remember to take the entrance marked "west" on the expressway to get to the doctor's office.

_____

_____

_____

2. You want to remember the year you retired, which is 1990.

_____

_____

_____

3. You want to remember Rose Campbell's name.

_____

_____

_____

4. You want to remember the name "Turner Medical Clinic."

_____

_____

_____

See page 131 for possible answers.

Visualization: Visualize a Picture of What You Want to Remember.

You have often heard that a picture is worth a thousand words. Visualization is the process of consciously creating an image in your mind of a task, a number, a name, a word, or a thought. If you take the time to translate words into a meaningful picture and then hold that picture in your mind for a few seconds, you are more likely to remember the name, the task, or the thought.

This technique can be used to remember such things as

- items you need to buy at the grocery store
- the route from the airport terminal to where you parked your car
- the laundry basket you want to bring up from the basement
- the name of a new breakfast cereal you want to try
- the punchline of a joke you recently heard

EXAMPLES

Estelle: When I was shopping last month, I saw such a beautiful dress in the window of a new store called Toshiros. I knew I'd never remember the name of this shop because it was unfamiliar to me, and I didn't know what it meant. When I repeated the name over to myself, I imagined a big hairy toe and a razor getting ready to shear the hair off—"Toe-shear-o."

Sue: I love to tell my friends about my favorite restaurant. It's so expensive that I can only go there once a year, so I don't see the name very often. It's called Justine's, which is a name I have trouble remembering. However, I do know that they have a young chef, so I imagine a very youthful face with a big chef's hat on, and think, "Why, he's 'just a teen.'"

Henry: I get so angry when I get up from my chair, put on my coat, walk to the back of my yard to get something from the garage, and then forget what I went to get. After taking a memory course, I found out that, if I take the time to picture what I'm getting up for, I can usually remember. Just yesterday, I wanted the flashlight from my car. I remembered it as blue, and I envisioned myself using it to look in the attic. When I got to the car, I had no trouble remembering what I had come to find.

EXERCISE: *VISUALIZATION*

Create a visual image to help you remember the following:

1. Mrs. Hammerman's name

_____

_____

_____

2. A car whose model name is Accord

_____

_____

_____

3. Parkinson's disease

_____

_____

_____

4. Lane 5B in a parking lot

_____

_____

_____

5. To buy a new windshield wiper blade while at the gas station

_____

_____

_____

See page 131 for possible answers.

Active Observation: Actively Observe and Think about What You Want to Remember.

It's often difficult to remember things you haven't observed clearly or with much interest. Active observation is the process of consciously paying attention to the details of what you see, hear, or read. By using active observation you can find meaning and vibrancy in a photograph, a new face, a nature scene, a conversation, an occurrence on the street, or a piece of artwork. Active observation contrasts with a passive attitude of letting life go on around you without much thought or interest. To actively observe a subject, think about the meaning of the subject, how you feel about it, how it affects you, and whether you want to remember it. Ask yourself questions that will reinforce its meaning. One key to remembering is being interested.

This technique can be used to remember such things as

- the design of a quilt you saw in a store
- how to play a new game your friend is teaching you

- the faces of people you see in the hallway of your apartment complex
- the difference between a fir tree and a juniper

EXAMPLES

Li Ming: I have very bad arthritis and can't go out much. I was so bored—every day was just the same, and my memory was getting really bad. My daughter gave me a bird feeder for my birthday, and little by little I started watching the birds that came. One day I saw a bird I didn't recognize. I asked my daughter if she knew what it was. She didn't, either, but the next time she visited me, she brought a colored picture book of hundreds of birds and facts about them. When we looked up the bird, I was amazed at how many kinds there are in Michigan. That bird feeder has changed my life! I'm seeing and learning new things, and I'm surprised that I can really remember them.

Steve: I parked in a parking garage when going to a large shopping mall. There were several up and down ramps on each level and no letters or numbers designating the area in which I had parked. I realized that I could easily misplace my car. I carefully observed the route I took to the exit stairway and, when I got there, looked back to reinforce the image of the location of my car. When I returned several hours later, I had a strong memory of where my car was located and how to get there.

Anita: After taking a memory course and learning about active observation, I decided to give it a try. I went to our local museum and spent some time looking at a painting of two women by Monet. Instead of just glancing at the painting as I usually do, I looked at the details as well as the whole and asked myself some questions: Did I think it was pretty? What time of year was it? Did the women look happy or sad? What were they wearing? Was there anything especially unusual about the painting? Would I like to have it in my living room? When I left the museum, I knew that I would remember something from this trip to the museum; it would not be just the usual blur of pictures.

EXERCISE: *ACTIVE OBSERVATION*

Look at the picture below, consciously paying attention to the details. Ask yourself questions about the picture's meaning and its effect on you as you look at it.

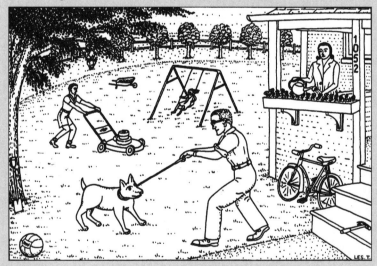

Now, cover the picture and see if you can answer these questions:

How many people are in the picture?
What is the boy doing?
What is the woman doing?
What is leaning against the house?
What is on the steps?
What is the number on the house?
What is the boy wearing?
What is the man doing?

If you are able to answer most of the above questions, you have used excellent powers of observation.

Elaboration: Elaborate on the Details of the Information You Want to Remember.

A brief, unexamined thought is very fragile and easily forgotten. When we elaborate on the details of a thought or idea, we encode it more deeply. We experience this depth of processing unintentionally when something very interesting or controversial occurs, such as a fist-fight at a basketball game. In our minds, we comment on the occurrence; we try to understand what happened; we relate it to what we know of the situation; we ask ourselves how we feel about it. This process can be used intentionally as a strategy for encoding information we want to remember.

Try this technique if you want to remember such things as

- the instructions for using your new vacuum attachments
- the platforms of the two mayoral candidates
- the courses that your grandson is taking in college

- the directions to the new recreation building
- the plot of a book you want to discuss with a friend

EXAMPLES

Manuel: I recently purchased a new VCR, read the instructions, and tediously followed them to record my favorite TV show. The next time I tried to record a show, I couldn't remember what to do and had to reread the instruction manual. Because I wanted to be able to program my VCR without referring to the manual, I was determined to encode the information well by using the technique of elaboration. I talked myself through the steps, figuring out the order and importance of each step. I translated the stilted manual directions into my own words. I repeated the steps several times to fix them in my long-term memory. I discovered that it works even better if you say the words aloud. After using elaboration, I could still remember the steps, even after being on vacation for three weeks.

Jill: I took the trip of a lifetime to the Hawaiian Islands. I visited three of the islands—all of which are gorgeous, yet different from each other. I wanted to be able to tell my friends about the islands without mixing them up. I had read in the newspaper that if you elaborate on the details of what you want to remember, you will encode the information more deeply. I thought about the different physical characteristics of the island, what I did on each island, and where I stayed. I made some associations between these details and the names of the islands. For several days I repeated these details, and now I find it easy to remember.

EXERCISE: *ELABORATION*

Every state has a nickname by which it is known. Here are the nicknames of three states:

Minnesota: The Gopher State
Missouri: The Show Me State
Montana: The Treasure State

See if you can use elaboration to encode these states and their nicknames so that you can remember them tomorrow. When you wake up tomorrow, ask yourself if you can remember this information. If not, try elaborating on it more fully.

16 You Do Not Have to Keep Everything in Your Head

Although there are times when you have to rely on your mind for remembering, most people use external reminders to prompt them throughout their daily lives. For example, you may use an alarm clock to wake up in the morning, keep a calendar of appointments, make grocery lists, use a kitchen timer for baking cookies, and use a marked pill box. You probably agree that there is no need to trust your memory in these situations. If you can use something in your environment to cue you, your mind is free to think of other things. Even though the following three external techniques may be familiar to you, consider finding new ways to adapt them to your needs.

Written Reminders: Write Things Down.

Although people of all ages use lists, calendars, appointment books, and notes to keep track of what they want to remember, some older people wonder whether written reminders are a crutch for a poor memory. On the contrary, writing things down is one of the most useful memory tools. As you age you may need to make even greater use of written reminders both for future events and as a diary of the day's happenings. If you want to remember these kinds of things better, record all information in one notebook.

The following list will give you ideas for creatively using written reminders.

- Keep a running list of things you need to do. As soon as you think of something, add it to the list. Keep this list in a permanent place where you can't help but notice it.
- Use an appointment book or calendar to remind yourself of calls you want to make in the future, such as phoning a friend after an operation. Make a habit of looking at your calendar frequently.
- Keep a list of health questions you want to ask your physician at your next appointment. Write down instructions from the physician before you the leave the office.
- Keep a diary of what has happened each day. Then, if you wonder whether you've written a letter or made an important phone call, you can refer to the diary. Include the names of people you've met.
- Keep a list of books you want to read or books you have read.
- Record letters and greeting cards sent and received.
- Record the name and dosage of each of your medications. Include the date you began taking it.
- Make lists of people whose names you want to remember, such as neighbors, members of a social group, or children of your friends.
- Record the anniversaries of events you would like to recall, such as the death of your friend's husband or child.
- Collect take-out menus from your favorite restaurants and mark your favorite menu items so you can recall what you enjoyed (or disliked) in the past.

ASSIGNMENT

Within the next three days, buy a notebook that you will use to record whatever you might want to remember. Keep a record for one week.

For example:

Diary

2004
Paid car insurance, 6/29
sent package to Jane, 7/1
7/4 met new neighbor—Jack

To Do List

Buy thread
Call plumber   769-1130
watch TV special
on S. Africa   9:00

Auditory Reminders: Use Sound to Trigger Your Memory.

Alarm clocks and timers can be used to remind yourself of something that can't be done immediately but that must be done at a specific time. A telephone answering machine can also be used to provide an auditory cue. Here are some examples of ways to use auditory reminders.

- If you make a phone call and get a busy signal, set your timer to remind yourself to call again.
- If you're busy writing letters and want to be sure to leave for an appointment at a specific time, set a portable timer and carry it with you to your desk.
- If you are away from home and want to remember to do something when you return, leave yourself a message on your answering machine.

Environmental Change: Change Something in Your Surroundings So It Jogs Your Memory.

One of the best and easiest ways to remind yourself of a specific task is to change something in your environment so that you notice the change. It then serves as a cue to jog your memory. It is imperative that you make the change as soon as you think of the task. Here are some examples of environmental cues that would jog your memory.

- Put the clothes to take to the cleaners in front of the door.
- Put a note on the kitchen table so you'll see it when you eat breakfast and remember to send a card to your son.
- Put a note on the steering wheel to remind yourself to vote or stop at the hardware store.
- Tie a string around the handles of your purse so you can't open it without being reminded to mail the letter that's inside.
- When you're down the basement, put an empty box in front of the stairway to remind yourself to turn off the electric heater before you go upstairs.

- Change your watch or ring to the other hand; you will constantly feel it. As you drive to your friend's house, it will remind you to tell him about the change in plans for the weekend. If you say aloud, "Tell Mario about the change in plans," the technique will work even better.

When using any of these external reminders, it is crucial to avoid procrastination. As soon as you think of something you need to do in the future, choose one of these techniques and act on it. If you think, "I'll add potatoes to my grocery list when this TV show is over," you may have forgotten all about the potatoes ten minutes later.

EXERCISE: *ENVIRONMENTAL CHANGE*

Think of ways to jog your memory for the following tasks by using environmental change.

1. You want to remember to return the coffeemaker to the office tomorrow.

_____

_____

_____

2. You are out grocery shopping and want to remember to call your dentist when you get home.

_____

_____

_____

3. You are at your exercise class and a friend asks you to bring a certain book to tomorrow's class.

_____

_____

_____

4. You want to remember to put out the garbage tomorrow.

_____

_____

_____

5. You are sitting in a meeting and you remember that you have to stop at the store on your way home.

_____

_____

_____

See page 132 for possible solutions.

17 Did I or Didn't I?

Many daily tasks are done automatically; we don't pay much attention to them. If you worry about whether you have unplugged the iron, turned off the electric blanket, or locked the door, you can use the technique of self-instruction.

Self-Instruction: Give Yourself Verbal Instructions about What You Want to Remember.

Use this technique to fix in your mind tasks about which you may ask yourself later, "Did I remember to do that?" As you turn off the coffeepot, say aloud to yourself, "I am now turning off the coffeepot," and you won't wonder about it later. This technique is powerful because it focuses your attention on a task that is often done automatically and thus is easily forgotten.

Sometimes you can use self-instruction to remind yourself to do something in the immediate future. You might need to provide more detail to reinforce your memory for a future task. As you drive to the grocery store at dusk, remind yourself aloud to turn off the headlights. One sentence is not enough in this case. You might say, "I'm putting my lights on as I go to the grocery store. When I get into the parking lot at Supermart, I must remember to turn them off." You might also visualize the lights shining on the store window as you arrive and then see yourself turning them off.

EXAMPLE

Dhara: One thing I hoped to get out of a memory course was learning how to remember whether I put detergent in the washer. I would get upstairs and have to go back down to the basement because I was never sure whether I had done it. The instructors suggested that, as I add the detergent, I say to myself, "There, I just put the soap into the washer." I gave it a try, and now I always say something aloud like "Good, I won't have to come down here again because I just added the soap," and it really works for me.

ASSIGNMENT

For the rest of the day, use self-instruction whenever you perform a task that might cause you to ask later, "Did I do that?" At the end of the day, look through the list below and check the ways you used this technique or might use it in the future. Notice whether using this technique was helpful.

turning off the stove/iron/coffeepot/heater
locking the door
turning off the car lights
turning down the heat

adding the laundry soap
releasing the emergency brake
taking medicine
turning off the basement light or front porch light
closing the garage door
putting the gas cap back on the gas tank
watering the plants

18 Remembering More Than One Item

The more items you have to remember, the harder it is. It is always easier to remember fewer items than more. There are techniques that can help when you have several items to remember. Look for ways to connect or combine items so they can be remembered collectively. You'll understand this concept after you read about the following techniques.

The Story Method: Devise a Story That Will Connect Things You Want to Remember.

The story method is the process of making up a simple, yet colorful, tale connecting items that seem to have no connection. Many people resist this technique because it seems either silly or too complicated. We believe that, if you give it a try, you will find it amazingly effective. This technique can be used to remember such things as

- two phone calls that you need to make when you get home
- three things you want to tell your daughter when you call her
- three items you need to pick up at the hardware store
- two books you want to get at the library

EXAMPLES

You wake up in the night and start thinking of what you need to do the next day. You want to remember that you need to call your dentist, return a rug to the department store, and buy filters for the furnace, but you don't want to get out of bed to write a list. You make up a story connecting these items by visualizing your **dentist** using a **rug** to keep himself warm because his **furnace** broke down.

You have to go to the cleaners and post office before you go home. You might make up a story about putting your **pants** into the **mailbox** and the chaos that would follow.

EXERCISE: *THE STORY METHOD*

Make up a one- or two-sentence story connecting the following items.

1. Getting a duplicate key made, picking up a birthday cake, and going to the bank

_____

_____

_____

2. Shopping for stationery, cologne, and a broom

_____

_____

_____

See page 132 for possible solutions.

Chunking: Chunk Individual Numbers into a Group.

We all know it's difficult to remember long numbers. When you are trying to remember a group of numbers, look for ways to combine them. This technique can be used to remember such things as

- phone numbers
- street addresses and zip codes
- Social Security and driver's license numbers

EXAMPLES

If you want to remember a local telephone number, such as 663-4735, you can group the seven numbers into four chunks, 66-34-7-35, which are easier to remember.

A driver's license or Social Security number has standard groupings, such as 343-49-4296. This number may be easier to remember if you change the "chunks" into 3-43-49-42-96 or 34-34-94-29-6 or 343-494-296.

EXERCISE: *CHUNKING*

Memorize your driver's license number or Social Security number by chunking the individual numbers. Analyze the sequence to see which way of chunking makes the most sense.

First-Letter Cues: Group the First Letters of a Series of Items.

This technique involves using the first letters of a list of words to form either another word or a meaningful sentence whose words begin with the same letters as the words on the list. Although this technique is hard to describe, it's easy to use. The following examples should give you the idea.

EXAMPLES

If you want to remember the names of the five Great Lakes, you can take the first letter of each lake and create the word HOMES (Huron, Ontario, Michigan, Erie, Superior).

If you want to remember the names of each of the presidents from Nixon to Bush, you can take the first letter of each name and form a sentence that has meaning to you. One example is: "Nine furry cats ran behind a cow barn" (Nixon, Ford, Carter, Reagan, Bush, Clinton, Bush).

You are in your car and think of four items you want from the grocery store but have no paper to write them on. You need butter, apples, a lemon, and milk. By rearranging the first letters of these four items, you find that you can form the word "lamb," which will serve as a memory cue. If the items do not form a word, try making a sentence with matching first letters. For example, if your list is soup, chicken, soap, and lettuce, you could create the sentence "Some cooks like soup" (or "Some chickens like soap!").

EXERCISE: *FIRST-LETTER CUES*

1. Create a word or sentence out of the first letters of the names of these downtown streets to help you remember the order. In this case, it's important to keep the letters in the same order as the streets.

Main
Adams
Lincoln
Rose
Brown

2. Try using this technique to remember the names of your friend's cats.

Radar
Alice
Chloe

See page 132 for possible solutions.

Create a Word: Expand Random Letters into a Familiar Word.

Sometimes you need to remember a group of letters that make no inherent sense, for example, license plates or business names. In this case you can add more letters, often vowels, to form a familiar word.

EXAMPLES

On a license plate, you might make the word "extra" out of "xra" or "lefty" out of "lft."

If you have trouble remembering the name of the company that manages your apartment building, PND, expand these letters to form the word "panda."

EXERCISE: *CREATE A WORD*

Expand the following letters into words:

1. PLM _____

2. RBT _____

3. GLW _____

4. STR _____

5. HLD _____

See page 132 for possible solutions.

Categorization: Group a List of Items by Category.

Categorization is the process of looking at a random list of items and seeing how to group them by category. It is easier to remember three categories that serve as cues for the nine items in the list than to remember each of the nine items separately.

EXAMPLE

These nine items could be grouped into three categories:

| popcorn | tuna | chips | pop | applesauce |
| cookies | juice | peas | milk | |

Canned goods: peas, applesauce, tuna
Snacks: popcorn, chips, cookies
Liquids: milk, juice, pop

EXERCISE: *CATEGORIZATION*

Categorize the following items:

broom	feather duster	Scotch tape
envelopes	dish soap	glue
sponge	furniture polish	bleach

_____

_____

_____

See page 133 for possible solutions.

19 Improving Your Ability to Recall

Often you might wish there was something that could help you recall well-known information when you need it. When you know that the information you want is in your long-term memory, but you can't recall it when you need it, there are three techniques you will find helpful.

Cue Yourself: Search Your Memory Bank for Related Facts That May Serve as Cues.

When you can't think of something that you know is in your long-term memory, merely thinking longer and harder may not work. However, there is a technique that is often useful. When you want to retrieve specific information from long-term memory, try thinking of related facts that might serve as cues to trigger the information you want.

This technique can be used for recalling

- the name of a famous person
- the French word for "friend"
- the name of a TV show
- how to get somewhere you haven't been for a long time
- the state in which the Grand Canyon is located

EXAMPLES

Vera was on her way to the video store to rent a movie she had seen many years ago. She thought she would recognize the title in the drama section of the video store. When she got there, she discovered that there were hundreds of titles in that section, all organized alphabetically. Rather than spend her time working her way from A to Z in this section, she thought, "I should be able to come up with this title." She began to search for cues that would trigger the name of the movie. She thought about who played the leading role and remembered Meryl Streep. She thought, "It took place in Africa . . . Of course! It's called 'Out of Africa.'"

Anna: My daughter lives in a new subdivision in town with a name I have trouble remembering. I wanted to tell my neighbor, but I didn't want to bother my daughter at work. I thought, "Maybe if I think of some related information, it will help." I could remember my daughter's address: 272 Appomattox. I thought about the entry sign to the subdivision, which has a cannon on it. "It must have something to do with the Civil War." It came to me—Gettysburg!

EXERCISE: *CUE YOURSELF*

See if you can recall the two candidates who ran for president of the United States in 1980. If you don't immediately know, search your memory for related facts that could serve as cues for this information.

See page 133 for the answer.

Alphabet Search: Go through the Alphabet to Jog Your Memory.

Alphabet search is the process of thinking through the sounds of the letters of the alphabet from A to Z to see if one will serve as a cue to jog your memory.

EXAMPLES

If you're trying to remember the name of someone you have just met, run through the sounds of the alphabet. Hearing the sound of the letter "m" may trigger the name Marian.

You want to describe the food you ate last night to a friend but can't remember the word "fettucini." You might go through the alphabet hoping that the beginning sound of one of the letters will cue your memory.

Review in Advance: Review in Advance What You May Be Called upon to Remember.

Everyone knows the feeling of forgetting familiar information, such as a friend's name or a well-known author. When you have to recall this type of information on demand, it sometimes takes a few seconds to bring it to mind—just long enough to cause a mental block. This experience is especially likely if you are asked to recall something or someone you haven't thought about for a while. When you know you will be called upon to remember certain names or information, reviewing ahead of time will often eliminate this problem.

This technique can be used to help you keep in mind

- the names of the grandnieces and grandnephews you will be seeing tomorrow
- the history of your medical problems when you see your doctor
- things you want to ask your grandson when you take him out to lunch
- the names of people you will be seeing at the annual meeting of your condominium association

EXAMPLES

If you are afraid you will not remember people's names at a family reunion or church social, prepare ahead of time by going over a list of everyone who might attend. Writing down the names and saying them aloud is more effective than simply reading through a list. As you say the name, visualize the person and something special about him or her, like red hair or a great laugh.

If you are going to a meeting of your book club, record the title of the book, the author, the names of characters, and your feelings about the book, and review your notes before you go.

If you are going to lunch with a friend, review the names of your friend's children and what you know about them beforehand so you can talk about them easily.

ASSIGNMENT

Think of the next group meeting you will attend (exercise class, senior center lunch group, bridge club, temple group), or try to think of the names of the people who live near you. List the names below and review them several times. If you have trouble listing all of them at one time, add to the list as the names come to you.

_____

_____

_____

_____

_____

_____

_____

_____

_____

_____

After you attend the meeting, consider whether the review helped you remember the names more easily. Did this technique work for you?

20 General Tips for Remembering

1. **Believe in yourself.** Don't let negative expectations defeat you. If you expect to fail, you won't even try. If you find yourself thinking, "I can't remember names," substitute "I may forget some names, but by using memory improvement techniques I can do better."

2. **Make conscious choices about what you want to remember.** No one can remember everything. So put effort and energy into those areas that are most important to you.

3. **Focus your attention on what you really want to remember.** Much of what is called "forgetting" is a lack of attention. Before you blame your memory, ask yourself if you were really paying attention.

4. **Cut out distractions.** Keep in mind that, as you age, you may find it more difficult to pay attention to more than one thing at a time. Recognize the limitations of working memory, and cut out distractions whenever possible.

5. **Give yourself plenty of time.** People of all ages forget more frequently when they are rushing. In general, if you have enough time to think about what you need to accomplish, you are less likely to forget something. You may also find that you need more time for learning new information and for recalling information from long-term memory. Give

yourself a little additional time and see if it helps in encoding and retrieving information.

6. **Use all of your senses.** Use as many senses as possible when you want to remember something well. When you say something aloud, you hear the sound. When you write something down, you see the words. If you want to remember the size or shape of something, use your sense of touch. Smell and taste are very powerful in triggering memories from long ago.

7. **Be organized.** The old saying "A place for everything, and everything in its place" is good advice for memory improvement. Make a decision to improve your organizational skills in whatever ways are important to you. If you routinely put your keys, glasses, purse, and bills in the same place, you will not waste time searching for them.

8. **Recognize and deal with the factors that may be negatively affecting your memory.** In this book, we have discussed factors that can affect the memory process for people of all ages. As you grow older, you may experience more of these negative influences. Think about which factors might be affecting your memory, and look for possible solutions or ways to compensate.

9. **Relax.** Tension interferes with the memory process; relaxing often lets the memory come to the surface. When you feel anxious about the possibility of forgetting, you may become preoccupied with the anxiety and unable to concentrate on recalling the needed information. The solution is to take a deep breath and relax; frequently the information will come to you.

10. **Laugh.** Laughter breaks the tension of forgetting and keeps a memory lapse in perspective. When you start to tell a friend about a book you are reading and can't remember the title, when you begin to introduce your niece and can't come

up with her name, admit that the word or name just escaped your mind, and laugh. Everyone has had that experience and can empathize.

11. **Enjoy past memories.** Recognize the richness of your storehouse of memories. You can experience great pleasure from recalling the events and people that have made up the fabric of your life. Life review can put the past and present into perspective. Take pride in your ability to remember the past and make it come alive for yourself and others.

Appendix: Alzheimer's Disease and Related Dementias

About Alzheimer's Disease

Alzheimer's (AHLZ-high-merz) disease is a progressive brain disorder that gradually destroys a person's memory and ability to learn, reason, make judgments, communicate, and carry out daily activities. As Alzheimer's progresses, individuals may also experience changes in personality and behavior, such as anxiety, suspiciousness, or agitation, as well as delusions or hallucinations.

Causes of Alzheimer's Disease

Alzheimer's disease has no known single cause, but in the last fifteen years scientists have learned a great deal about factors that may play a role.

Late-onset Alzheimer's, which chiefly affects individuals over age sixty-five, is the more common form of the illness that is most often associated with the term "Alzheimer's disease." The greatest known risk factors for late-onset Alzheimer's are increasing age and a family history of the disease. The likelihood of developing late-onset Alzheimer's approximately doubles every five years after age sixty-five. By age eighty-five, the risk reaches nearly 50 percent. Scientists have thus far discovered one gene that increases the risk for late-onset disease.

Rare, familial types of Alzheimer's found in a few hundred families worldwide have been linked to specific genes. Individuals who inherit these genes are virtually certain to develop the disease, usually before age sixty-five and sometimes as early as their thirties or forties.

Researchers worldwide are working to discover other factors that affect Alzheimer risk. Some of the most exciting preliminary evidence suggests that strategies for generally healthy aging may also reduce the risk of developing Alzheimer's. These measures include controlling blood pressure, weight, and cholesterol levels; exercising both body and mind; and staying socially active.

What is the difference between Alzheimer's disease and normal age-related memory difficulties?

Activity	A Person with Memory Problems	A Person with Normal Age-Associated Memory Changes
forgets	whole experiences	parts of an experience
remembers later	rarely	often
can follow written or spoken directions	gradually unable	usually able
can use notes	gradually unable	usually able
can care for self	gradually unable	usually able

Source: *Caring for People with Alzheimer's Disease: A Manual for Facility Staff,* by Lisa P. Gwyther (Washington, D.C.: American Health Care Association and Alzheimer's Association, 2001).
Note: Determination of whether memory loss is associated with Alzheimer's disease can only be made by health care professionals.

How Does Alzheimer's Disease Affect the Brain?

Scientists believe that whatever triggers Alzheimer's disease begins to damage the brain years before symptoms appear. When symptoms emerge, nerve cells that process, store, and retrieve information have already begun to degenerate and die. Scientists regard two abnormal microscopic structures called "plaques" and "tangles" as the hallmarks of Alzheimer's disease. Amyloid plaques (AM-uh-loyd plaks) are clumps of protein fragments that accumulate outside of the brain's nerve cells. Tangles are twisted strands of another protein that form inside brain cells. Scientists have not yet determined the exact role that plaques and tangles may play.

Diagnosing Alzheimer's Disease

Although Alzheimer's symptoms can vary widely, the first problem that many people notice is forgetfulness severe enough to affect performance at home, at work, or in favorite activities. Sometimes the decline in memory may be more obvious to a family member or close friend than to the affected individual. Other common symptoms include confusion, getting lost in familiar places, and difficulty with language. The Alzheimer's Association encourages everyone who notices these symptoms in themselves or someone close to them to consult a physician.

A skilled physician can diagnose Alzheimer's disease with 90 percent accuracy. Because there is no single test for Alzheimer's, diagnosis usually involves a thorough medical history and physical examination as well as tests to assess memory and the overall function of the mind and nervous system. The physician may ask a family member or close friend about any noticeable change in the individual's memory or thinking skills.

One important goal of the diagnostic workup is to determine whether symptoms may be due to a treatable condition. Depression, medication side effects, certain thyroid conditions, excess use of alcohol, and nutritional imbalances are all potentially treatable disorders that may sometimes impair memory or other mental functions. Even if the diagnosis is Alzheimer's, timely identification enables individuals to take an active role in treatment decisions and planning for the future.

Alzheimer's is the leading cause of dementia, a group of conditions that all gradually destroy brain cells and lead to progressive decline in mental function. Most diagnostic uncertainty arises from occasional difficulty distinguishing Alzheimer's disease from one of these related disorders.

Other Causes of Dementia

Vascular dementia, also known as multi-infarct dementia, results from brain damage caused by multiple strokes (infarcts) within the brain. Symptoms can include disorientation, confusion, and behavioral changes. Vascular dementia is neither reversible nor curable, but treatment of underlying conditions such as high blood pressure may sometimes slow progression.

Normal pressure hydrocephalus (NPH) is a rare disease caused by an obstruction in the flow of spinal fluid leading to a buildup of fluid in the brain. Symptoms include difficulty in walking, memory loss, and incontinence. NPH may be related to a history of meningitis, encephalitis, or brain injury and is occasionally correctable with surgery.

Parkinson's disease affects the control of muscle activity, resulting in tremors, stiffness, and speech difficulties. In late stages, dementia can occur. Parkinson's drugs can improve steadiness and control but have no effect on mental deterioration.

Dementia with Lewy bodies is a disorder that, although progressive, is often initially characterized by wide variations in attention and alertness. Affected individuals often experience visual hallucinations as well as muscle rigidity and tremors similar to those associated with Parkinson's disease.

Huntington's disease is a fatal, progressive hereditary disorder characterized by irregular movements of the limbs and facial muscles, a decline in thinking ability, and personality changes.

Frontotemporal dementia, also known as Pick's disease, is a rare brain disease that closely resembles Alzheimer's, with personality changes and disorientation that may precede memory loss.

Creutzfeldt-Jakob disease (CJD) is a rare, ultimately fatal disorder of infectious or genetic origin that typically causes memory failure and behavioral changes. A recently identified form called "variant Creutzfeldt-Jakob disease (vCJD)" is the human disorder thought to be caused by eating meat from cattle affected by "mad cow disease" (bovine spongiform encephalopathy). vCJD tends to appear in much younger individuals than those affected by sporadic or inherited Creutzfeldt-Jakob.

Treating Alzheimer's Disease

Alzheimer medication approved by the U.S. Food and Drug Administration (FDA) may temporarily delay memory decline for some individuals, but none of the currently approved drugs is known to stop the underlying degeneration of brain cells. Certain drugs approved to treat other illnesses may sometimes help with the emotional and behavioral symptoms of Alzheimer's.

One important part of treatment is supportive care that helps individuals and their families come to terms with the diagnosis, obtain information and advice about treatment options, and maximize quality of life through the course of the illness.

As the pace of research accelerates, scientists funded by the Alzheimer's Association, the pharmaceutical industry, universities, and our federal government have gained detailed understanding of the basic disease process at work in the Alzheimer brain. Experts believe that several of these processes may offer promising targets for a new generation of treatments to prevent, slow, or even reverse damage to nerve cells.

About the Alzheimer's Association

For more than twenty years, the Alzheimer's Association has provided reliable information, created supportive programs and services for families, increased resources for dementia research, and influenced changes in public policy. We are the world leader in Alzheimer research and support. Our goal is to create a powerful constituency of passionate Americans that places the prevention and cure of Alzheimer's disease at the top of its agenda. To learn more, please contact us:

Contact Center: 800-272-3900

TDD Access: 312-335-8882

Web site: www.alz.org

e-mail: info@alz.org

What Additional Resources Are Available?

The following resource materials are available from your local chapter or the national office of the Alzheimer's Association:

About Alzheimer's Disease

About the Alzheimer's Association

Is it Alzheimer's? Warning Signs You Should Know

Steps to Getting a Diagnosis: Finding Out if It's Alzheimer's Disease

Steps to Enhancing Communication: Interacting with Persons with Alzheimer's Disease

Steps to Understanding Challenging Behaviors: Responding to Persons with Alzheimer's Disease

Steps to Planning Activities: Structuring the Day at Home

Steps to Understanding Legal Issues: Planning for the Future

Steps to Enhancing Your Home: Modifying the Environment

Caregiver Stress: Signs to Watch For, Steps to Take

The 36-Hour Day: A Family Guide to Caring for Persons with Alzheimer Disease, Related Dementing Illnesses, and Memory Loss in Later Life by Nancy L. Mace, M.A., and Peter V. Rabins, M.D., M.P.H. Baltimore: Johns Hopkins University Press, 1999 (third edition)

Drug Fact Sheets

Answers to the Exercises

Recall (page 18) and Recognition (page 23)

1. Springfield
2. Judy Garland
3. Iwo Jima
4. Spiro Agnew

Understanding the Memory Process (pages 24–25)

When you go to the library and notice a lot of colorful books on the "new books" shelf, you are using **sensory memory.** You read through the titles and think about whether they interest you. These conscious thoughts occur in a component of memory called **working memory.** Then you notice a book by a favorite author, John Grisham. You take down the book, notice how long it is, read the dust jacket, and decide that you don't have time to read it this month. This process is called **encoding.** The information about the book leaves your conscious thought and goes into the component of memory called **long-term memory**, where it may be available for **retrieval** at another time. When you get home, you notice another of Grisham's books in your den. This favorite book serves as a **cue** to remind you of the book in the library. The connection between the library book and your book at home is called **association.**

How Memory Works (page 25)

1. F
2. F
3. T
4. T
5. T
6. T
7. F

Learning New Information (pages 36–38)

1. People who are depressed or anxious.
2. One example of a distorted thought is "I am worthless."
3. A depressed person is less likely to be active.
4. One problem-solving strategy is to break problems into small steps.

How Memory Changes (page 42)

1. F
2. F
3. T
4. T
5. F
6. T

Factors That Affect Memory (pages 76–77)

1. T
2. F
3. T
4. F
5. T
6. T
7. F
8. T
9. F
10. T

Association (pages 86–87)

1. Since you are going to the doctor, associate "west" with "wellness"—both words begin with W.
2. Associate 1990 with the fact that you've always said you'd like to celebrate your ninetieth birthday.
3. Associate "Campbell" with Campbell's soup and "Rose" with the red of the label on the soup can.
4. Associate the name "Turner" with turning your health around. Say to yourself several times, "Turner turned my health around."

Visualization (pages 89–90)

1. Visualize a giant hammer hitting a man.
2. Imagine your car being towed with a cord.
3. Visualize a woman sitting in the park with the sun beating down on her shoulders.
4. Visualize five Balloons tied to your car antenna.

5. Visualize yourself paying for a tank of gas and asking the attendant for a replacement windshield wiper.

Environmental Change (pages 100–101)

1. Put the coffeemaker in front of the door as soon as you think about returning it.
2. Write yourself a note in big letters on the grocery bag so that when you unpack the groceries you'll see it.
3. Tie a string around your purse handle or wrist. When you get home you will be reminded to get the book out. Be sure to put it with your exercise clothes or equipment.
4. Put a big sign on the bathroom mirror or front door.
5. Change your watch or ring to the other hand.

The Story Method (page 106)

1. Envision a birthday cake shaped like a safe. You use a key to open it and find a huge pile of money.
2. See yourself breaking the bottle of cologne and sweeping up the pieces into a box of stationery.

First-Letter Cues (page 109)

1. Mother Always Liked Rose Best.
2. CAR or ARC

Create a Word (page 110)

1. plum
2. robot
3. glow

4. string
5. hold

Categorization (page 111)

Desk items	Cleaning tools	Cleaning products
envelopes	sponge	dish soap
Scotch tape	broom	furniture polish
glue	feather duster	bleach

Cue Yourself (page 113)

Jimmy Carter and Ronald Reagan

Recommended Reading

Barry Gordon. *Intelligent Memory: Improve the Memory That Makes You Smarter.* New York: Viking, 2003.

Cynthia R. Green. *Total Memory Workout: Eight Easy Steps to Maximum Memory Fitness.* New York: Bantam, 1999.

Gary Small. *The Memory Bible: An Innovative Strategy for Keeping Your Brain Young.* New York: Hyperion, 2002.